T0226955

Cognitive Behavioral Therapy for Anxiety and Depression

Editors

STEFAN G. HOFMANN
JASPER A.J. SMITS

PSYCHIATRIC CLINICS OF NORTH AMERICA

www.psych.theclinics.com

December 2017 • Volume 40 • Number 4

ELSEVIER

1600 John F. Kennedy Boulevard • Suite 1800 • Philadelphia, Pennsylvania, 19103-2899

http://www.theclinics.com

PSYCHIATRIC CLINICS OF NORTH AMERICA Volume 40, Number 4
December 2017 ISSN 0193-953X, ISBN-13: 978-0-323-55296-7

Editor: Lauren Boyle
Developmental Editor: Kristen Helm

Psychiatric Clinics of North America (ISSN 0193-953X) is published quarterly by Elsevier Inc., 360 Park Avenue South, New York, NY 10010-1710. Months of issue are March, June, September, and December. Business and Editorial Offices: 1600 John F. Kennedy Blvd., Suite 1800, Philadelphia, PA 19103-2899. Periodicals postage paid at New York, NY and additional mailing offices. Subscription prices are $303.00 per year (US individuals), $628.00 per year (US institutions), $100.00 per year (US students/residents), $369.00 per year (Canadian individuals), $460.00 per year (international individuals), $791.00 per year (Canadian & international institutions), and $220.00 per year (Canadian & international students/residents). Foreign air speed delivery is included in all *Clinics'* subscription prices. All prices are subject to change without notice. **POSTMASTER:** Send address changes to *Psychiatric Clinics of North America*, Elsevier Health Sciences Division, Subscription Customer Service, 3251 Riverport Lane, Maryland Heights, MO 63043. **Customer Service: 1-800-654-2452 (US). From outside the United States, call 1-314-447-8871. Fax: 1-314-447-8029. E-mail: journalscustomerservice-usa@elsevier.com (for print support)** and **journalsonline support-usa@elsevier.com (for online support).**

Reprints. For copies of 100 or more, of articles in this publication, please contact the Commercial Reprints Department, Elsevier Inc., 360 Park Avenue South, New York, New York 10010-1710. Tel.: 212-633-3874, Fax: 212-633-3820, E-mail: reprints@elsevier.com.

Psychiatric Clinics of North America is covered in *MEDLINE/PubMed (Index Medicus), Current Contents/Social and Behavioral Sciences, Social Science Citation Index, Embase/Excerpta Medica,* and PsycINFO.

Contributors

EDITORS

STEFAN G. HOFMANN, PhD
Professor of Psychology, Department of Psychological and Brain Sciences, Boston University, Boston, Massachusetts, USA

JASPER A.J. SMITS, PhD
Department of Psychology, Institute for Mental Health Research, The University of Texas at Austin, Austin, Texas, USA

AUTHORS

GERHARD ANDERSSON, PhD, Dr Med Sci
Professor, Department of Behavioural Sciences and Learning, Linköping University, Linköping, Sweden; Department of Clinical Neuroscience, Karolinska Institute, Stockholm, Sweden

NICOLE R. BROWNFIELD, BSc (Hons)
Cognitive Behavior Therapy Research Unit, School of Psychological Sciences, Monash Institute of Cognitive and Clinical Neurosciences, Monash University, Melbourne, Australia

PER CARLBRING, PhD
Professor, Department of Psychology, Stockholm University, Stockholm, Sweden

RIANNE A. DE KLEINE, PhD
Institute of Psychology, Leiden University, Leiden, The Netherlands

ANDREW J. FLIGHTY, BPsychSc
Cognitive Behavior Therapy Research Unit, School of Psychological Sciences, Monash Institute of Cognitive and Clinical Neurosciences, Monash University, Melbourne, Australia

ANGELINA F. GÓMEZ, BA
Doctoral Student in Clinical Psychology, Department of Psychological and Brain Sciences, Boston University, Boston, Massachusetts, USA

DEVON E. HINTON, MD, PhD
Associate Professor, Department of Psychiatry, Massachusetts General Hospital, Harvard Medical School, Boston, Massachusetts, USA

STEFAN G. HOFMANN, PhD
Professor of Psychology, Department of Psychological and Brain Sciences, Boston University, Boston, Massachusetts, USA

CARLY JOHNCO, PhD
Postdoctoral Research Fellow, Centre for Emotional Health, Department of Psychology, Macquarie University, Sydney, New South Wales, Australia

NIKOLAOS KAZANTZIS, BA(Hons), MA, PGDipClinPsych, PhD, FAPS
Associate Professor, Program Director, Clinical Psychology, Director, Cognitive Behavior Therapy Research Unit, School of Psychological Sciences, Monash Institute of Cognitive and Clinical Neurosciences, Monash University, Melbourne, Australia

MICHAEL E. LEVIN, PhD
Faculty, Department of Psychology, Utah State University, Logan, Utah, USA

TANIA M. LINCOLN, PhD
Professor and Head of Working Group, Clinical Psychology and Psychotherapy, Institute of Psychology, Universität Hamburg, Hamburg, Germany

LIVIA MOSELY, BEng, BA, PDM
Cognitive Behavior Therapy Research Unit, School of Psychological Sciences, Monash Institute of Cognitive and Clinical Neurosciences, Monash University, Melbourne, Australia

PETER J. NORTON, PhD
Professor, School of Psychological Sciences, Monash University, Clayton, Victoria, Australia

ELLA L. OAR, PhD
Postdoctoral Research Fellow, Centre for Emotional Health, Department of Psychology, Macquarie University, Sydney, New South Wales, Australia

THOMAS H. OLLENDICK, PhD
Distinguished Professor, Department of Psychology, Child Study Center, Virginia Polytechnic Institute and State University, Blacksburg, Virginia, USA

SANDRA M. OPOKA, MSc
Doctoral Student, Clinical Psychology and Psychotherapy, Institute of Psychology, Universität Hamburg, Hamburg, Germany

ANUSHKA PATEL, MA
Department of Psychology, The University of Tulsa, Tulsa, Oklahoma, USA

MARK B. POWERS, PhD
Department of Psychology, Institute for Mental Health Research, The University of Texas at Austin, Austin, Texas, USA; Baylor University Medical Center, Baylor T. Boone Pickens Cancer Hospital, Dallas, Texas, USA

PASQUALE ROBERGE, PhD
Associate Professor, Department of Family Medicine and Emergency Medicine, Faculty of Medicine and Health Sciences, Université de Sherbrooke, Sherbrooke, Québec, Canada

JASPER A.J. SMITS, PhD
Department of Psychology, Institute for Mental Health Research, The University of Texas at Austin, Austin, Texas, USA

DAVID F. TOLIN, PhD
Director, Anxiety Disorders Center, The Institute of Living, Adjunct Professor of Psychiatry, Yale School of Medicine, Hartford, Connecticut, USA

MICHAEL P. TWOHIG, PhD
Faculty, Department of Psychology, Utah State University, Logan, Utah, USA

ALEXSANDRA S. USATOFF, BSc, GDipPsych, GDipProfPsych
Cognitive Behavior Therapy Research Unit, School of Psychological Sciences, Monash Institute of Cognitive and Clinical Neurosciences, Monash University, Melbourne, Australia

AMY WENZEL, PhD, ABPP
Wenzel Consulting, LLC, Perelman School of Medicine, University of Pennsylvania, Bryn Mawr, Pennsylvania, USA

Contents

Cognitive behavioral therapy's main strategies are active, problem focused, and collaborative. Cognitive restructuring is a strategy in which clinicians help patients to identify, evaluate, and modify inaccurate or otherwise unhelpful thinking associated with emotional distress. Behavioral activation provides a framework for patients, particularly those who are depressed, to increase engagement in activities that provide a sense of accomplishment or pleasure. The goal of exposure is for anxious patients to experience an extinction of fear by having planned contact with feared stimuli and situations. Problem solving allows patients to systematically approach and address their life problems by using cognitive and behavioral techniques.

This article reviews the extant literature on mediators of change in cognitive behavioral therapy (CBT) for anxiety and depression. The authors briefly discuss the efficacy of CBT for anxiety and depression and methods of mediation analysis and detection. Then the authors discuss fear extinction in anxiety treatment and cognitive change in depression treatment.

Treatment adherence has posed a substantial challenge not only for patients but also for the health profession for many decades. The last 5 years have witnessed significant attention toward adherence with cognitive behavioral therapy (CBT) homework for anxiety and depressive disorders, and adherence assessment methods have diversified. However, there remains a large component of the adherence process not assessed in CBT, with patient effort, engagement, and the known role for treatment appraisals and beliefs necessitating the pursuit of improved adherence assessment methods.

Depression and anxiety are prominent comorbid disorders in psychosis and relevant to psychotic symptom formation and maintenance, which poses the question of whether psychological interventions are effective in improving symptoms of depression and anxiety in patients with psychosis. A systematic review of the literature identified 14 studies evaluating a broad range of interventions targeting depression, anxiety, and posttraumatic stress disorder in patients with psychosis. The reviewed studies support the effectiveness of cognitive behavioral interventions in improving the target symptoms. Further research is needed to examine whether the effects carry over to psychotic symptoms in the long term.

Anxiety and depression are highly prevalent disorders in youth. Assessments for these disorders in young people typically include clinician-administered instruments, such as diagnostic interviews and parent- and youth-report questionnaires. Cognitive behavioral therapy is considered a well-established treatment for both anxiety and depression. Latest research in the field is exploring innovative methods to enhance treatment outcome and improve access to evidence-based treatments.

Transdiagnostic cognitive behavioral (CBT) therapy is a modified form of CBT designed to be applicable with patients across the range of anxiety and related emotional disorders. Based on emerging genetic, neurologic, developmental, cognitive, and behavioral science, transdiagnostic CBT may alleviate barriers to dissemination and accessibility by providing a single treatment approach across diagnoses. Data from clinical trials and meta-analyses suggest treatment efficacy that is comparable with traditional CBT approaches, with possibly superior efficacy among patients with multiple comorbid anxiety and emotional diagnoses. Limitations in the evidence base and remaining areas for future research are discussed.

Internet-assisted cognitive behavioral therapy (ICBT) is a way to deliver cognitive behavioral therapy (CBT) that has been found to generate similar effects as face-to-face CBT in some studies. Results have been replicated by different research groups. This article presents the treatment format and reviews evidence for mood and anxiety disorders. Future developments are discussed, including the lack of theories specific for the treatment format and ways to handle comorbidity. Although some programs have been implemented, there is a need for further studies in clinical settings. Overall, clinician-assisted ICBT is becoming one of the most evidence-based forms of psychological treatment.

In increasingly multicultural societies, cognitive behavioral therapy (CBT) must be made appropriate for diverse groups. This article examines cultural adaptations of CBT, focusing on anxiety and depressive disorders. The article presents a culturally informed, transdiagnostic model of how anxious-depressive distress is generated and culturally shaped. Guided by this model, it discusses how interventions can be designed to decrease anxiety-type and depressive-type psychopathology in a culturally sensitive way. It describes such concepts as explanatory model bridging, cultural grounding, and contextual sensitivity.

The present meta-analysis examined controlled trials of pharmacologic augmentation of cognitive behavioral therapy (CBT) for patients with anxiety or depressive disorders. The additive effect of medications was small for both anxiety and depressive disorders at posttreatment, and there was no additive benefit after medications were discontinued. A small body of evidence suggested that antidepressant medications are an efficacious second-line treatment for patients failing to respond to CBT alone. In anxiety disorders, novel agents thought to potentiate the biological mechanisms of CBT showed small effects at posttreatment; after discontinuation, some of these agents were associated with an increasing effect.

This article reviews the ways in which mindfulness practices have contributed to cognitive and behavioral treatments for depression and anxiety. Research on mindfulness-based interventions (MBIs) has increased rapidly in the past decade. The most common include mindfulness-based stress reduction and mindfulness-based cognitive therapy. MBIs are effective in reducing anxiety and depression symptom severity in a range of individuals. MBIs consistently outperform non–evidence-based treatments and active control conditions, such as health education, relaxation training, and supportive psychotherapy. MBIs also perform comparably with cognitive behavior therapy (CBT). The treatment principles of MBIs for anxiety and depression are compatible with standard CBT.

Acceptance and commitment therapy (ACT) is a modern form of cognitive behavioral therapy based on a distinct philosophy and the basic science of cognition. This article reviews the core features of ACT's theoretic model of psychopathology and treatment and its therapeutic approach. It provides a systematic review of randomized controlled trials (RCTs) evaluating ACT for depression and anxiety disorders. Summarizing 36 RCTs, ACT appears to be more efficacious than waitlist conditions and treatment-as-usual, with largely equivalent effects relative to traditional cognitive behavioral therapy. Evidence indicates that ACT treatment outcomes are mediated through increases in psychological flexibility, its theorized process of change.

PSYCHIATRIC CLINICS OF NORTH AMERICA

THE CLINICS ARE AVAILABLE ONLINE!
Access your subscription at:
www.theclinics.com

Preface

The Evolution of Cognitive Behavioral Therapy for Anxiety and Depression

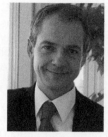 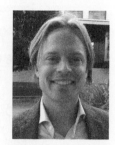

Stefan G. Hofmann, PhD   Jasper A.J. Smits, PhD
Editors

Cognitive behavioral therapy (CBT) identifies a family of treatment protocols describing evidence-based strategies for overcoming mental health problems. A review of the empirical literature identified 269 meta-analytic studies examining CBT for nearly every psychiatric problem.[1] A summary of the various CBT protocols can easily fill a 3-volume textbook series.[2] Although the specific treatment strategies differ depending on the specific target problems, they all share a common scientific foundation.[3]

Clearly, CBT has become one of the big success stories of contemporary psychiatry. Soon after the generic CBT model was formulated by Aaron T. Beck[4] and others, it revolutionized the field of psychiatry. In recognition of his contribution, Dr Beck received the Lasker Award in 2006, a highly prestigious medical prize. Lasker jury appropriately described this therapy approach as one of the most important advances, if not the most important advance, in the treatment of mental disorders.[5]

Despite its success, CBT has not yet reached its full potential. As is true for any scientific enterprise, CBT has been evolving over the years. Over the years, this family of interventions has evolved from a diverse set of specific treatment strategies for single DSM-defined pathologies toward treatments targeting core processes involved in treatment change.[6] As this focus on core processes strengthens, the emphasis on syndromes will likely weaken in the near future.[7]

Focused on two of the most common mental health problems, this issue will first review basic CBT strategies (Amy Wenzel), some core mechanisms (Mark B. Powers, Rianne A. de Kleine, and Jasper A. J. Smits), and the use of homework in CBT (Nikolaos Kazantzis, Nicole R. Brownfield, Livia Mosely, Alexsandra S. Usatoff, and Andrew J. Flighty). This is followed by articles on CBT for anxiety and depression in severe mental disorders (Sandra M. Opoka and Tania M. Lincoln) and in children and

Psychiatr Clin N Am 40 (2017) xi–xii
http://dx.doi.org/10.1016/j.psc.2017.08.011
0193-953X/17/© 2017 Published by Elsevier Inc.

adolescents (Ella L. Oar, Carly Johnco, and Thomas H. Ollendick). Some of the contemporary and likely future applications include transdiagnostic/unified treatment for anxiety disorders (Peter J. Norton and Pasquale Roberge), Internet-assisted CBT (Gerhard Andersson and Per Carlbring), cultural adaptations (Devon E. Hinton and Anushka Patel), pharmacological enhancements (David F. Tolin), mindfulness-based approaches (Stefan G. Hofmann and Angelina F. Gómez), and acceptance and commitment therapy (Michael P. Twohig and Michael E. Levin). We believe this issue provides a representative cross-sectional snapshot of the current state of CBT for two of the most common mental health problems.

Stefan G. Hofmann, PhD
Department of Psychological and Brain Sciences
Boston University
648 Beacon Street, 6th Floor
Boston, MA 02215, USA

Jasper A.J. Smits, PhD
Department of Psychology
University of Texas at Austin
305 East 23rd Street, Stop E9000
Austin, TX 78712, USA

E-mail addresses:
shofmann@bu.edu (S.G. Hofmann)
smits@utexas.edu (J.A.J. Smits)

REFERENCES

1. Hofmann SG, Asnaani A, Vonk JJ, et al. The efficacy of cognitive behavioral therapy: a review of meta-analyses. Cognit Ther Res 2012;36:427–40.
2. Hofmann SG, editor. The Wiley handbook of cognitive behavioral therapy, vols. I–III. Chichester (United Kingdom): John Wiley & Sons, Ltd; 2014.
3. Hofmann SG, Asmundson GJ, Beck AT. The science of cognitive therapy. Behav Ther 2013;44:199–212.
4. Beck AT. Cognitive therapy and the emotional disorders. New York: Guilford University Press; 1975.
5. Altman LK. Psychiatrist is among five chosen for medical award. New York Times 2006. Available at: http://www.nytimes.com/2006/09/17/health/17lasker.html. Accessed September 8, 2017.
6. Hayes SC, Hofmann SG, editors. Process-based CBT: the science and core clinical competencies of cognitive behavioral therapy. Oakland (CA): New Harbinger; 2017.
7. Hayes SC, Hofmann SG. The third wave of CBT and the rise of process-based care. World Psychiatry, in press.

Basic Strategies of Cognitive Behavioral Therapy

Amy Wenzel, PhD, ABPP

KEYWORDS

- Strategy • Cognitive restructuring • Behavioral activation • Exposure
- Inhibitory learning • Problem solving

KEY POINTS

- Cognitive behavioral therapy is an active, strategic, and time-sensitive psychotherapeutic intervention.
- Cognitive restructuring helps patients to identify, evaluate, and modify maladaptive thoughts and beliefs associated with emotional distress.
- Behavioral activation helps patients to increase engagement in activities that provide a sense of accomplishment and pleasure.
- Exposure allows anxious patients to have systematic contact with feared stimuli and situations, overcoming avoidance and reliance on ritualistic behavior to neutralize anxiety.
- Problem solving teaches patients systematic skills for addressing life problems and overcoming unhelpful attitudes about problems.

BASIC STRATEGIES OF COGNITIVE BEHAVIORAL THERAPY

Cognitive behavioral therapy (CBT) is an active, problem-focused, and time-sensitive approach to treatment that aims to reduce emotional distress and increase adaptive behavior in patients with a host of mental health and adjustment problems. Cognitive behavioral therapists deliver interventions in a strategic manner, such that interventions (1) emerge from the customized case formulation of the patient's clinical presentation, (2) are delivered in a collaborative manner with the patient, (3) are designed to move patients forward and directly toward meeting their treatment goals, and (4) are seen through in their entirety so that their efficacy can be evaluated with "data" collected by the patient.[1] Thus, the basic strategies of CBT are efficient, focused, and targeted.

Disclosures: None.
Wenzel Consulting, LLC and University of Pennsylvania School of Medicine, 1062 Lancaster Avenue, Suite #24, Bryn Mawr, PA 19010, USA
E-mail address: awenzel@dramywenzel.com

Historically, the focus of CBT has been on two psychological domains: cognition and behavior. According to the theory that underlies CBT, maladaptive or unhelpful cognition lies at the heart of understanding psychopathology.[2] Patients with depression, for example, are often characterized by a "negative cognitive triad," such that they have negative beliefs about themselves, the world, and the future that reinforce and perpetuate their mood disturbance.[3] It follows then, that a basic cognitive strategy in CBT would be to help patients modify such negative thinking as a vehicle to improve their mood. Today, this strategy, called *cognitive restructuring*, is a central one in the delivery of CBT, although it should be noted that contemporary off-shoots of CBT promote alternative cognitive approaches, such as distancing from thoughts rather than changing them.[4] Behavioral strategies in CBT are focused on overcoming avoidance, engaging in prosocial behavior, and achieving self-care. For example, *behavioral activation* for depression helps patients to become more actively engaged in their lives, whereas *exposure* for anxiety, obsessive-compulsive and related, and trauma- and stressor-related disorders helps patients to extinguish fear responses by having systematic contact with feared stimuli and situations. Moreover, most patients who present for treatment are dealing with an array of life problems, so a *problem-solving* strategy can be adopted using cognitive techniques to help patients view problems in an adaptive manner and behavioral techniques to allow them to implement solutions to their problems. Although there are many additional strategies used by cognitive behavioral therapists, these four, cognitive restructuring, behavioral activation, exposure, and problem solving, are among the strategies that are most fundamental to this work and are those that are discussed in this article.

COGNITIVE RESTRUCTURING

Cognitive restructuring is the process by which clinicians help patients to recognize, evaluate, and if necessary, modify maladaptive or otherwise unhelpful thinking. Cognitive behavioral therapists apply cognitive restructuring to situation-specific thoughts that arise in times of stress or adversity (called *automatic thoughts*) as well as to negative underlying beliefs. Consider a patient who describes an upsetting incident in which her son was not invited to another child's birthday party. She reports the automatic thoughts, "This is my fault. The child's mother does not like me." Not surprisingly, she experiences a host of negative emotions, including guilt, shame, and sadness. A cognitive behavioral therapist would use cognitive restructuring to help her understand the role that her thinking plays in her negative affect, consider other reasons why her son might not have been invited to the party, recognize that her son is invited to many other birthday parties, and evaluate how catastrophic this situation truly is. The cognitive behavioral therapist would also be alert to themes in the automatic thoughts that would signify a negative underlying belief, such as "I'm undesirable" or "I'm unlikable." The therapist would then work, over time, to shift that negative belief to one that is more reasonable and balanced (eg, "I'm just as likable as everyone else."). This section describes three steps for implementing cognitive restructuring, as well as several specific techniques and tools to achieve cognitive restructuring's aim of modifying maladaptive or otherwise unhelpful thinking.

Identifying Maladaptive Thinking

Most cognitive behavioral therapists begin by focusing cognitive restructuring of automatic thoughts, and over time, they use this work to develop hypotheses about the nature of underlying beliefs that would benefit from cognitive restructuring later in the course of treatment. To identify automatic thoughts, cognitive behavioral therapists ask their patients questions such as, "What was running through your mind in that situation?" and "What did that situation mean to you?" Although these questions seem straightforward, it takes many patients practice to move beyond mere description of the situation (eg, "My son will not join his friends at the party.") or a surface-type reaction that cannot easily be reframed (eg, "What is going on here?") to the fundamental meaning that accounts for the greatest variance of their emotional distress (eg, "This is my fault. The child's mother does not like me."). Cognitive behavioral therapists work with patients in session to identify automatic thoughts associated with upsetting situations that they have recently experienced, and patients are encouraged to continue this practice between sessions by recording, prospectively, upsetting situations, automatic thoughts, and accompanying emotional reactions.

As mentioned previously, underlying beliefs can often be discerned by examining the themes that pervade automatic thoughts. Automatic thoughts that reflect themes of social rejection are often associated with beliefs like "I'm undesirable," "I'm unlikable," or "I'm unlovable." Automatic thoughts that reflect themes of personal shortcomings are often associated with beliefs like "I'm inadequate" or "I'm a failure." Automatic thoughts that reflect a sense of self-deprecation are often associated with beliefs like "I'm worthless" or "I'm a burden." Automatic thoughts that reflect a sense of threat are often associated with beliefs like "I'm vulnerable," "I can't cope," and "The world is dangerous." In addition to examining themes associated with automatic thoughts, cognitive behavioral therapists also use the *downward arrow technique* to identify underlying beliefs,[5] such that they probe the meaning associated with automatic thoughts several times until there is no meaning that is more fundamental than that which has been identified. For example, in the case that is being followed to this point, the cognitive behavioral therapist might ask, "What would it mean if the mother doesn't like you?" The patient might respond with, "It means that my son and I won't have many friends." The therapist might further respond with, "What would it say about you that you have few friends?" The patient might respond with a statement that points to the underlying belief, "I'm totally undesirable. No one likes me." Cognitive behavioral therapists are also alert to instances in which patients demonstrate significant affect while engaging in cognitive restructuring (eg, tearfulness, shaking, aversion of eye contact), as displays of affect often indicate that a patient has arrived on a powerful and upsetting underlying belief.

Evaluating Maladaptive Thinking

Cognitive behavioral therapists do not automatically assume that their patients' thinking is dysfunctional; rather, they encourage their patients to critically evaluate their thinking to ensure that it is as accurate and balanced as possible. The most common way to evaluate maladaptive thinking is to use *Socratic questioning*, or open-ended questions that allow patients to examine all sides of their thinking and draw conclusions about its accuracy and helpfulness. The delivery of Socratic questions facilitates the process of *collaborative empiricism*, in which the therapist and patient, together, take a scientific approach to examining the patient's thinking and draw conclusions on the basis of the evidence or "data" collected.

Any question can be posed to evaluate maladaptive thinking in the spirit of collaborative empiricism; because each patient's thinking style is unique, no two courses of Socratic questioning to achieve the aims of cognitive restructuring will look alike. One of the most common lines of questioning used by cognitive behavioral therapists is to ask patients to examine the factual evidence that does and does not support the thoughts and beliefs that they have identified. In many instances, patients find that there is very little factual evidence that supports the thinking that is associated with emotional distress. *Reattribution* is a Socratic technique in which patients consider the wide array of explanations for an upsetting event that they experienced, rather than focusing solely on something being wrong with them or something bad that they did. Patients who struggle with anxiety can be asked about the best, worst, and most likely outcomes of situations in which they perceive threat, with the idea that in most instances, the most likely outcome is much more closely aligned with the best that can happen than with the worst that can happen. These patients also can contemplate how bad the worst-case outcome would truly be and how they would cope if it indeed occurred. Patients who have trouble distancing themselves from their thinking about an upsetting situation can be asked what they would tell a friend in that situation, as in many instances, what they would tell a friend is very different than what they are saying to themselves. To evaluate the helpfulness of their thinking, patients can consider the advantages and disadvantages of holding onto their thoughts and beliefs or the effects of continuing to think as they are versus changing their thinking.

These Socratic questions can be used in the service of belief modification as well as the modification of automatic thoughts. However, belief shift tends to occur more gradually over time, so the evaluation of underlying beliefs usually occurs over the course of several sessions. One way to achieve this aim is to encourage patients to maintain a *positive data log*, such that they, prospectively, record events and occurrences from their lives that support a new, more balanced belief. It is hoped that the accumulation of evidence that supports the new belief will facilitate critical evaluation of the degree to which the old belief is truly accurate. Belief modification also can be achieved by powerful in-session experiential techniques, such as when patients conduct a role-play in which they, at their current age, impart wisdom on themselves at key times in their younger years when maladaptive underlying beliefs were being formed. Patients who participate in these exercises often learn that negative experiences that happened to them were not due to personal defects, but rather to circumstances beyond their control and that they were quite adept at surviving those experiences.

Modifying Maladaptive Thinking

If, on the basis of Socratic questioning, patients conclude that their thinking is inaccurate or otherwise unhelpful, cognitive behavioral therapists work with them to develop an *adaptive response*, or a new, more balanced statement that takes into account the data that emerge from questioning. The adaptive response is not merely a simply platitude like "Everything will be OK," as such a statement would likely not be believable in times of emotional distress. Instead, the adaptive response is often several sentences long, addressing the array of evidence inconsistent with the original automatic thought, the other explanations for an upsetting situation, the likelihood of a worst-case scenario, the specific way in which the patient would cope with a worst-case scenario, and so on. Effective adaptive responses are those that are associated with a significant reduction in associated emotional distress, relative to the original automatic thought, and are compelling and believable enough that they reduce emotional distress in subsequent instances in which the original automatic thought is again identified. Underlying beliefs that are ultimately modified are done so after the application of several belief modification techniques across the course of several sessions.

Tools and Techniques

Perhaps the most well-known tool to facilitate cognitive restructuring is the *thought record*, which, in its original form, is a sheet of paper with columns in which patients record a few words about upsetting situations that they experienced in their lives, the key associated automatic thought(s), and their emotional experiences (and the intensity of those emotional experiences). Over time, thought records become more elaborate, such that patients can record an adaptive response and the outcome of adopting the adaptive responses (eg, such as a reduction in emotional intensity; a different course of action that they would take). Patients complete entries on the thought record in session as they are acquiring skill in cognitive restructuring, and they maintain the thought record for homework between sessions.

Although many professionals believe that the thought record is synonymous with cognitive restructuring, or even with CBT, in reality, there are several other tools that facilitate cognitive restructuring. In fact, in the age of technology, many patients prefer not to record their cognitive restructuring work on a sheet of paper (and find it to be cumbersome), and instead record their work on one of the many mobile phone applications available for this purpose. Other patients, such as those who are suicidal or those with panic disorder, experience episodes of intense affect that narrow their attention on their symptoms and interfere with their ability to apply systematic logic and reason.[6,7] It is difficult for these patients to use a thought record in the times of distress that they most need to apply cognitive restructuring. In these cases, they can create *coping cards*, which are index cards or business cards that contain a recurrent automatic thought and a compelling, believable adaptive response that can be consulted in a time of need. Some patients report that they believe adaptive responses "intellectually," but that they do not believe them "emotionally." In these cases, they can work with their therapist to devise a *behavioral experiment*, such that they design a way to "test" a negative prediction that they are making in their own environment, such as by testing out whether they will truly be rejected by someone with whom they would like to spend more time. Moreover, the goals of cognitive restructuring can be achieved simply through conversation between the patient and the cognitive behavioral therapist in session.

Efficacy

Surprisingly, there is a paucity of research on the efficacy of cognitive restructuring alone; it is usually evaluated in the context of full CBT treatment packages, of which it is one significant component. One exception[8] demonstrated that for every standard deviation increase in the use of Socratic questioning with any one depressed patient, there is a corresponding decrease of approximately 1.5 points on the Beck Depression Inventory-II[9] completed at the time of the subsequent session. Moreover, research on the broader approach of cognitive reappraisal, or a strategy in which people reinterpret the meaning of a stimulus to alter their emotional response,[10] suggests that it is successful in reducing negative affect in experimental settings.[11,12] However, there is evidence that full packages of CBT, including cognitive restructuring, are no more effective than two of the behavioral strategies described in the subsequent sessions: (1) behavioral activation,[13,14] and (2) exposure.[15] Cognitive behavioral therapists are encouraged to implement cognitive restructuring when it is indicated on the basis of the individualized formulation of the patient's clinical presentation and to conduct themselves as "scientist-practitioners," gathering "data" on the efficacy of cognitive restructuring over time to verify their inclusion in a cognitive behavioral treatment package for any one patient.

BEHAVIORAL ACTIVATION

Peter Lewinsohn's[16] behavioral theory of depression was developed in the 1970s, around the same time as Aaron T. Beck's cognitive therapy. According to Lewinsohn's behavioral theory, depression can be explained by a lack of response-contingent positive reinforcement in one's life. This means that the patients are receiving little reward from their environment, particularly reward that is obtained by their own efforts. As a result, depressed individuals often retreat, isolate themselves, and report a sense of helplessness. *Behavioral activation* is a behavioral CBT strategy that helps patients to actively reengage in their lives by doing things that allow them to take care of themselves; contribute to their families, their professions, and society at large; and bring them a sense of accomplishment and pleasure.

Lewinsohn and Graf[17] developed a behavioral treatment for depression based on these principles, and A. T. Beck and colleagues[3] included behavior modification into his now classic CBT treatment manual for depression. However, the term "behavioral activation" was not used until the late 1990s, when Neil Jacobson and his colleagues[13] evaluated the only the behavioral component of CBT for depression (ie, behavioral activation) with the behavioral activation plus cognitive restructuring of automatic thoughts and with a full CBT package, consisting of behavioral activation, cognitive restructuring of automatic thoughts, and cognitive restructuring of beliefs. Results from their research, as well as an impressive follow-up clinical trial in which the full behavioral activation intervention was manualized,[14] demonstrated that behavioral activation is regarded as just as potent a treatment for depression as is a full package of CBT. In this section, I describe two components of behavioral activation that were included in the earliest CBT packages for depression, and I then elaborate on additional specific techniques incorporated into contemporary behavioral activation protocols.

Activity Monitoring

Activity monitoring refers to an exercise in which patients track the activities in which they engage every hour for the period between sessions. In addition to recording their activities, they rate the degrees of mastery (or sense of accomplishment) and pleasure that they obtain from these activities. At the end of the day, patients provide an overall rating of their level of depression. It is expected that patients will observe an inverse association between the degree of mastery and pleasure they obtain from their activities and their level of depression for the day, which will serve as an impetus for reengaging in more meaningful activities in their lives.

Activity Scheduling

Patients use the results from activity monitoring to determine days and times in their lives in which they could stand to work in activities associated with a greater sense of mastery or pleasure (which would, in turn, be expected to life mood and have an antidepressant effect). *Activity scheduling* is a mechanism by which patients determine when they plan to engage in these activities. When patients make plans to schedule some activities associated with a sense of mastery or pleasure, they again track their activity level for the week, acknowledging the scheduled activities in which they engaged, rate the level of mastery and pleasure associated with their daily activities, and provide an overall rating of depression at the end of the day. It is expected that activity scheduling will yield an improvement in mood and that increased engagement will persist when patients observe the "data" that they collected, indicating that they feel better when they are more actively engaging in activities that give them a sense of mastery or pleasure.

Contemporary Techniques

In its contemporary framework, behavioral activation refers to a set of techniques that have been incorporated into treatment protocols in their own right, even without the cognitive components of CBT. However, behavioral activation is also incorporated into broader CBT packages for depression as well as CBT packages for other mental health disorders that are comorbid with depression.[18] Contemporary behavioral activation has its foundation in activity monitoring and scheduling, but it expands on these fundamental techniques significantly by adding a framework for overcoming avoidance, a focus on values, and tools for overcoming rumination (which often interferes with action).[19–22]

Cognitive behavioral therapists who practice contemporary behavioral activation pay close attention to the form and function, rather than content, of behavior. They are adept at identifying instances in which their patients' behavior is serving an avoidance function, rather than a more adaptive function. For example, a patient might report that she declined a social invitation to take care of herself, as she has had difficulty sleeping and is feeling especially stressed. Although, on the surface, this might seem like healthy self-care behavior, but if it serves the function of avoidance and isolation, preventing the patient from obtaining response-contingent positive reinforcement and feeding into a pattern that is making her depression spiral, then it is doing more harm than good. Not only do cognitive behavioral therapists attend to such contingencies in their patients' behavior, they also are cognizant of their own reactions in session to reinforce patients' reports of adaptive behavior, such as by providing encouragement when patients report a behavioral activation "victory." Throughout their work with patients, cognitive behavioral therapists conduct A-B-C analyses to understand the "a"ntecedents, "b"ehaviors, and "c"onsequences of behaviors that reinforce depression.

In addition, cognitive behavioral therapists who practice contemporary behavioral activation encourage their patients to clarify their values in many domains in their lives.[23,24] The idea is that patients will gain the greatest antidepressant benefit when they are behaving consistently with their values. Thus, patients can clarify how they want to act in major life domains, such as close relationships and their profession, and they can set tangible goals that will help to translate their values to meaningful behavior. They can then determine the behaviors they can commit to implementing on a regular basis to live their lives according to their values and achieved desired goals.

Efficacy

The data supporting behavioral activation's efficacy are impressive. Some randomized controlled trials obtained results indicating that behavioral activation was just as efficacious[13] or more efficacious[14] than a full package of CBT, with gains persisting a least two years following the completion of treatment.[25,26] Evidence for its efficacy has been extended to Latino patients,[27] patients with breast cancer and depression,[28] and smokers with elevated depressive symptoms.[29] Meta-analyses have yielded pre-post treatment effect sizes ranging from 0.78[30] to 0.87[31] and controlled posttreatment effect sizes ranging from 0.56 when compared with brief psychotherapy to 0.75 when compared with supportive psychotherapy.[32]

EXPOSURE

Exposure is defined as systematic contact with a feared stimulus or situation to facilitate extinction, or the reduction in the conditioned fear response to conditioned stimuli that represents threat.[33] It is a central strategy in the treatment of anxiety, obsessive-compulsive and related, and trauma- or stressor-related disorders. Exposure can take several forms. For example, *in vivo exposure* is actual contact with a feared stimulus or situation, such as when a person with a spider phobia allows a spider to crawl on her arm, or a person with contamination fears touches toilets and floors in public restrooms. *Imaginal exposure* is used when it is infeasible or unethical to simulate actual feared stimuli situations and is implemented when a patient imagines feared consequences of contact with the stimulus or situation, or constructs and reviews vivid narratives of worries about the future or past traumas. *Interoceptive exposure* is used for patients who are fearful of anxiety symptoms themselves (eg, in panic disorder, health anxiety) and involves the intentional evocation of those symptoms (eg, by spinning in a chair, by running up and down a flight of stairs). This section describes the implementation of exposure, as well as two theoretic frameworks that explain its mechanism of action.

Development of a Fear Hierarchy

A preliminary step in conducting exposure is to develop a *fear hierarchy*, or an ordered sequence of feared stimuli or situations. Patients work their cognitive behavioral therapist to identify an array of specific stimuli or situations that provoke a fear response, and they assign a subjective "units of discomfort" rating to each one (eg, 0 = no fear response; 10 = panic attack). The hierarchy is then ordered from the least fear-provoking to the most fear-provoking items, with the idea that patients will start at the beginning of the hierarchy and work up, in a graded fashion, to items that are higher on the hierarchy. However, it should be noted that empirical research has demonstrated that outcome is enhanced when patients choose random items on their hierarchy,[34] rather than proceeding in a systematic order, so cognitive behavioral therapists need not be limited to the sequence that is identified when the hierarchy is developed.

Implementation of Exposure

It is recommended that cognitive behavioral therapists conduct an exposure exercise in session, with the idea that patients complete similar exposure exercises most days outside of session for homework.[1] When cognitive behavioral therapists practice from the fear reduction perspective, they encourage their patients to remain in the exposure for as long as it takes for anxiety to dissipate (a phenomenon called *habituation*), without escaping. Exposure conducted from this framework often necessitates that sessions last longer than the traditional 45-minute or 50-minute psychotherapy session to achieve habituation. When practicing from this framework, it is expected that patients will achieve *within-session habituation*, or the decline in fear within a single, prolonged trial of exposure, and *between-session habituation*, or the decline in initial, peak, and ending fear ratings across trials of the same exposure exercise.

However, a critical review of the literature by Michelle Craske and her colleagues[35] found that there was, at best, weak evidence for these premises, and that many empirical studies found no association between within-session and between-session habituation and outcome. Instead, they proposed an *inhibitory learning* framework to explain the mechanism by which exposure works. According to this model, excitatory pathways are those in which the stimulus or situation is associated with an aversive outcome, and inhibitory pathways are those in which the stimulus or situation is no longer associated with an aversive outcome. From this perspective, exposure is successful when inhibitory pathways are strengthened, even if self-reported fear during and across exposures does not reliably decrease. What changes, instead, is the learning that occurs, such that patients' expectations for aversive outcomes are violated by participating in exposure. For example, if a patient believes that he can only tolerate the interoceptive exposure exercise of overbreathing for 30 seconds, and then engages in the exercise for 60 seconds, then he has learned that he can tolerate more contact with the feared situation than he an estimated.

Thus, cognitive behavioral therapists who practice from an inhibitory learning framework are mindful of several ways for patients to achieve the violation of their expectancies when participating in an exposure exercise.[35–37] First, they ask their patients to explicitly state their expectations for an aversive outcome from the exposure trial, and they structure the exposure in a way that patients have an experience that is different from the expectations that they specified. To further enhance learning, after encouraging their patients to engage in exposures to single cues, they combine cues to achieve *super-extinction* of the stimulus-fear association. For example, an obsessive-compulsive patient with contamination fears might simultaneously touch toilets and floors of a public restroom while simultaneously imagining catastrophic contamination of his family members. Reliance on safety signals and behaviors (eg, carrying a bottle of alprazolam, seeking reassurance) is discouraged, as it deprives patients of the opportunity to learn that aversive outcomes will not occur in the absence of the safety signal or behavior, or if they do, that the patient can tolerate them. Moreover, variation in exposures is strongly encouraged to achieve the consolidation and generalization of learning that occurs,[38] as fear responses are more likely to recur when people encounter a novel fearful stimulus in a context that is different from the one in which they practiced exposure. Cognitive behavioral therapists who deliver exposure from an inhibitory learning framework emphasize fear tolerance to a greater degree than fear reduction.

Efficacy

Like behavioral activation, a significant body of literature has demonstrated the efficacy of exposure for anxiety, obsessive-compulsive and related, and trauma- and stressor-related disorders. In one meta-analysis of exposure-based CBT for anxiety disorders, a very large pre-post-treatment effect size of 1.56 was observed.[39] Moreover, meta-analytic work has demonstrated that exposure-based CBT outperforms placebo-controlled conditions[40] and other credible treatments for anxiety disorders (eg, relaxation)[41] and that patients who complete a trial of exposure-based CBT score within one SD of the population norm on self-report inventories of anxiety.[42] However, these data are based on exposure delivered from a habituation framework, and full-scale randomized controlled trials examining the efficacy of inhibitory learning-based exposure and comparing exposure delivered from a habituation framework with exposure delivered from an inhibitory learning framework have yet to be conducted.

PROBLEM SOLVING

Intervention in the form of problem solving is a mainstay of CBT. Many clients present for treatment reporting that they are overwhelmed with the problems that they are facing in their lives. Because CBT is generally a present-focused and problem-focused approach to treatment, a central goal of CBT is to help clients identify and enact solutions to their problems. Of course, it is often the case that to enact a solution to a problem, a client must interact with others, such as asking questions to obtain information, asking for help, or setting boundaries. Thus, along with coaching in the acquisition of problem-solving skills, clients also can benefit from skills training to help them enact the solutions to their problems in the most effective way possible.

Problem-solving therapy is a cognitive behavioral problem-solving approach that has been in existence for more than 30 years[43–46] and, like behavioral activation, is a CBT treatment package in its own right, as well as an approach whose techniques are incorporated into broader packages of CBT. The most current edition of the problem-solving therapy manual[46] describes four "toolkits" that can be implemented on the basis of case formulation of the patient's clinical presentation. One toolkit includes techniques to apply when patients are overwhelmed with problem solving, including externalization (ie, writing down relevant information), visualization (ie, using mental imagery to achieve problem clarification and rehearsal of solution implementation), and simplification (ie, breaking the problem down into smaller pieces). The second toolkit includes skills for distress tolerance and stress management during problem solving to avoid engagement in self-defeating behaviors (eg, controlled breathing, muscle relaxation). The third toolkit describes cognitive techniques to modify a *negative problem orientation*, or a negative view of problems that interfere with motivation and follow-through (eg, "Problems are threats rather than opportunities"; "I'm a bad person because I am experiencing this problem.").

Problem-solving therapy's fourth toolkit forms the mainstay of the way in which cognitive behavioral therapists teach problem-solving skills to those patients who are characterized by deficits in this area. There are four steps to this planful, rational approach to problem solving. The first step of planful problem solving is *problem definition and formulation*, in which patients define their problems and requisite components, set goals for problem solving, and identify obstacles that might interfere with achieving those goals. Next, the *generation of alternatives* refers to brainstorming all possible solutions without judgment. Once patients have generated solutions to their problems, they turn to *decision making,* often using an *advantages-disadvantages analysis* to weigh the pros and cons of each proposed solution. A logical homework exercise for clients is to implement the solution that had been decided on. Thus, the fourth step of problem solving is *solution implementation and verification.* Verification refers to the fact that cognitive behavioral therapists invite their clients to discuss the implementation of their solution at the time of the next session so that they can evaluate whether it was successful and what was learned from the exercise.

Although there is a paucity of research that has evaluated the efficacy of problem solving as one strategy incorporated into a larger CBT package, a great deal of empirical support supports problem-solving therapy as a treatment package in the treatment of a host of mental health and adjustment problems, including (but not limited to) depression, anxiety, intellectual disability, cancer, diabetes, obesity, and chronic pain.[45,46] Results from meta-analyses suggest that problem solving is equally as efficacious as other bona fide treatments for mental health disorders and adjustment to medical illness[47] and that it is associated with moderate to large effect sizes in the treatment of depression.[48]

SUMMARY

CBT's active, problem-focused nature makes it highly efficacious in the treatment of a host of mental health and adjustment problems. Although this article describes four standard CBT strategies, cognitive restructuring, behavioral activation, exposure, and problem solving, it is important to recognize that cognitive behavioral therapists implement a wide array of strategic interventions on the basis of the case formulation of the patient's clinical presentation, the treatment goals, and the patient's preferences. For example, CBT experts are increasingly developing and adapting strategies that promote acceptance,[4] intervene at the level of emotional experiencing,[49,50] and harness the power of therapeutic relationship in facilitating change.[51] Future researchers are encouraged to isolate the efficacy of individual CBT strategies and the percentage of variance accounted by each of them in outcome associated with overall packages of CBT for mental health disorders.

REFERENCES

1. Wenzel A. Strategic decision making in cognitive behavioral therapy. Washington, DC: American Psychological Association; 2013.
2. Beck AT. Cognitive therapy: past, present, and future. J Consult Clin Psychol 1993;62:164–98.
3. Beck AT, Rush AJ, Shaw BF, et al. Cognitive therapy of depression. New York: Guilford Press; 1979.
4. Hayes SC, Strosahl KD, Wilson KG. Acceptance and commitment therapy: the process and practice of mindful change. 2nd edition. New York: Guilford Press; 2012.
5. Burns DD. Feeling good: the new mood therapy. New York: Signet; 1980.
6. Adler A, Jager-Hymen S, Green K, et al. Initial validation of the attentional fixation questionnaire for suicide attempts. Cogn Ther Res 2015;39:492–8.
7. Wenzel A, Sharp IR, Sokol L, et al. Attentional fixation in panic disorder. Cogn Behav Ther 2006;35:65–73.
8. Braun JD, Strunk DR, Sasso KE, et al. Therapist use of Socratic questioning predicts session-to-session symptom change in cognitive therapy for depression. Behav Res Ther 2015;70:32–7.
9. Beck AT, Steer RA, Brown GK. Beck depression inventory—second edition. San Antonio (TX): The Psychological Corporation; 1996.
10. Gross JJ. The emerging field of emotion regulation: An integrative review. Rev Gen Psychol 1998;2:271–99.
11. Denny BT, Ochsner KN. Behavioral effects of longitudinal training in cognitive reappraisal. Emotion 2014;14:425–33.
12. Diedrich A, Hofmann SG, Cuijpers P, et al. Self-compassion enhances the efficacy of explicit cognitive reappraisal as an emotion regulation strategy in individuals with major depressive disorder. Behav Res Ther 2016;82:1–10.
13. Jacobson NS, Dobson KS, Truax PA, et al. A component analysis of cognitive–behavioral treatment for depression. J Consult Clin Psychol 1996;64:295–304.
14. Dimidjian S, Hollon SD, Dobson KS, et al. Randomized trial of behavioral activation, cognitive therapy, and antidepressant medication with the acute treatment of adults with major depression. J Consult Clin Psychol 2006;74:658–70.
15. Hope DA, Heimberg RG, Bruch MA. Dismantling cognitive-behavioral group therapy for social phobia. Behav Res Ther 1995;33:637–50.
16. Lewinsohn PM. A behavioral approach to depression. In: Friedman M, Katz MM, editors. The psychology of depression: contemporary theory and research. New York: John Wiley and Sons; 1974. p. 157–85.
17. Lewinsohn PM, Graf M. Pleasant activities and depression. J Consult Clin Psychol 1973;41:261–8.
18. Wenzel A. Innovations in cognitive behavioral therapy: strategic interventions for creative practice. New York: Routledge; 2017.
19. Addis ME, Martell CR. Overcoming depression one step at a time: the new behavioral activation treatment to getting your life back. Oakland (CA): New Harbinger; 2004.
20. Dimidjian S, Barrera M Jr, Martell C, et al. The origins and current status of behavioral activation treatments for depression. Annu Rev Clin Psychol 2011;7:1–38.

21. Martell CR, Addis ME, Jacobson NS. Depression in context: strategies for guided action. New York: Norton; 2001.
22. Martell CR, Dimidjian S, Herman-Dunn R. Behavioral activation for depression: a clinician's guide. New York: Guilford Press; 2010.
23. Lejuez CW, Hopko DR, Hopko SD. A brief behavioral activation treatment for depression. Behav Modif 2001;25:255–86.
24. Lejuez CW, Hopho DR, Acierno R, et al. Ten year revision of the brief behavioral activation treatment for depression (BATD): revised treatment manual (BATD-R). Behav Modif 2011;35:111–61.
25. Gortner ET, Gollan JK, Dobson KS, et al. Cognitive behavioral treatment for depression. Relapse prevention. J Consult Clin Psychol 1998;66:377–84.
26. Dobson KS, Hollon SD, Dimidjian S, et al. Randomized trial of behavioral activation, cognitive therapy, and antidepressant medication in the prevention of relapse and recurrence in major depression. J Consult Clin Psychol 2008;76: 468–77.
27. Kanter JW, Santiago-Rivera AL, Santos MM, et al. A randomized hybrid efficacy and effectiveness trial of behavioral activation for Latinos with depression. Behav Ther 2015;46:177–92.
28. Hopko DR, Armento MEA, Robertson SMC, et al. Brief behavioral activation and problem solving therapy for depressed breast cancer patients: randomized trial. J Consult Clin Psychol 2011;79:834–49.
29. MacPerson T, Tull MT, Matusiewicz A, et al. Randomized controlled trial of behavioral activation smoking cessation treatment for smokers with elevated depressive symptoms. J Consult Clin Psychol 2010;78:55–71.
30. Mazzucchelli T, Kane R, Rees C. Behavioral activation treatments for depression in adults: a meta-analytic review. Clin Psychol Sci Prac 2009;16:383–411.
31. Cuijpers P, van Straten A, Warmerdam L. Behavioral activation treatments of depression: a meta-analysis. Clin Psychol Rev 2007;27:318–26.
32. Ekers D, Richards D, Gilbody S. A meta-analysis of randomized trials of behavioural treatment of depression. Psychol Med 2007;38:611–23.
33. Abramowitz JS, Deacon BJ, Whiteside SPH. Exposure therapy for anxiety: principles and practice. New York: Guilford Press; 2011.
34. Lang AJ, Craske MG. Manipulations of exposure-based therapy to reduce return of fear: a replication. Behav Res Ther 2000;38:1–12.
35. Craske MG, Kircanski K, Zelikowsky M, et al. Optimizing inhibitory learning during exposure therapy. Behav Res Ther 2008;46:5–27.
36. Abroamowtiz SJ, Arch JJ. Strategies for improving long-term outcomes in cognitive behavioral therapy for obsessive-compulsive disorder: insights from learning theory. Cogn Behav Prac 2014;21:20–31.
37. Craske MG, Treanor M, Conway CC, et al. Maximizing exposure therapy: an inhibitory learning approach. Behav Res Ther 2014;58:10–23.
38. Rowe MK, Craske MG. Effects of varied-stimulus exposure training on fear reduction and return of fear. Behav Res Ther 1998;36:719–34.
39. Norton PJ, Price ED. A meta-analytic review of adult cognitive-behavioral treatment outcome across the anxiety disorders. J Nerv Ment Dis 2007;195:521–31.
40. Powers MB, Halpern JM, Ferenschak MP, et al. A meta-analytic review of prolonged exposure for posttraumatic stress disorder. Clin Psychol Rev 2010;30: 635–41.
41. Siev J, Chambless DL. Specificity of treatment effects: cognitive therapy and relaxation for generalized anxiety and panic disorders. J Consult Clin Psychol 2007;75:513–22.

42. Abramowitz JS. Does cognitive behavioral therapy cure obsessive-compulsive disorder? A meta-analytic evaluation of clinical significance. Behav Ther 1998; 29:339–55.
43. D'Zurilla TJ. Problem solving therapy: a social competence approach to clinical intervention. New York: Springer; 1986.
44. D'Zurilla TJ, Nezu AM. Problem solving therapy: a social competence approach to clinical intervention. 2nd edition. New York: Springer; 1999.
45. D'Zurilla TJ, Nezu AM. Problem solving therapy: a positive approach to clinical intervention. 3rd edition. New York: Springer; 2007.
46. Nezu AM, Nezu CM, D'Zurilla TJ. Problem solving therapy: a treatment manual. New York: Springer; 2013.
47. Malouff JM, Thorsteinsson EB, Schutte NS. The efficacy of problem solving therapy in reducing mental and physical health problems: a meta-analysis. Clin Psychol Rev 2007;27:46–57.
48. Cuijpers P, van Straten A, Warmerdam L. Problem solving therapies for depression: a meta-analysis. Eur Psychiatry 2007;22:9–15.
49. Hofmann SG. Emotion in therapy: from science to practice. New York: Guilford Press; 2016.
50. Thoma NC, McKay S. Working with emotion in cognitive behavioral therapy: techniques for clinical practice. New York: Guilford press; 2015.
51. Kazantzis N, Dattilio FM, Dobson KS. The therapeutic relationship in cognitive-behavioral therapy: a clinician's guide. New York: Guilford Press; 2017.

Core Mechanisms of Cognitive Behavioral Therapy for Anxiety and Depression: A Review

Mark B. Powers, PhD[a,b,*], Rianne A. de Kleine, PhD[c], Jasper A.J. Smits, PhD[a]

KEYWORDS

- Anxiety • Depression • Mechanisms • Mediators • CBT • Review • Cognitive
- Behavioral

KEY POINTS

- Fear extinction is the type of learning that takes place during cognitive behavioral therapy (CBT) for anxiety.
- Inhibitory learning is a process by which fear extinction takes place.
- Cognitive change largely mediates CBT for depression in whatever manner it is achieved (through cognitive restructuring, behavioral activation, and so forth).

In this article, the authors seek to summarize the core mechanisms of cognitive behavioral therapies (CBTs). Core mechanisms of CBT include the specific psychological factors responsible for symptom improvement with therapy. The authors do not discuss nonspecific factors that can also be therapeutic, such as expectancy, credibility, and therapeutic alliance.[1] In addition, they do not cover neural mechanisms of change in this article. It is difficult to separate psychological and neural mechanisms because they may measure the same processes at different levels of analysis. However, work is underway to further delineate the role of the limbic system and the prefrontal cortex as explanatory mechanisms of psychological mediators of CBT.[2–8] The authors first briefly define CBT and mediators of change. Next, they discuss core

Conflicts of Interest and Source of Funding: Dr J.A.J. Smits is a paid consultant for Microtransponder, Inc. Dr M.B. Powers and Dr R.A. de Kleine have declared no competing interests. This study was funded by a grant from the National Institutes of Health (NIH; K01DA035930; R34MH099318; R34DA034658). NIH plays no role in approving the publications.
 a Department of Psychology, Institute of Mental Health Research, The University of Texas at Austin, 305 E. 23rd Street, Stop E9000, Austin, TX 78712, USA; b Baylor University Medical Center, T. Boone Pickens Cancer Hospital, 3409 Worth Street Tower, Suite C2.500, Dallas, TX 75246, USA; c Institute of Psychology, Leiden University, PO Box 9500, 2300 RA Leiden, The Netherlands
* Corresponding author. The University of Texas at Austin, 305 E. 23rd Street, Stop E9000, Austin, TX 78712.
E-mail address: mbpowers@utexas.edu

Psychiatr Clin N Am 40 (2017) 611–623
http://dx.doi.org/10.1016/j.psc.2017.08.010
0193-953X/17/© 2017 Elsevier Inc. All rights reserved.

mechanisms of change in CBT for anxiety and related disorders, including extinction and threat reappraisal. Finally, they cover cognitive change as the most researched mediator of CBT for depression.

CBTs are a family of treatments that share a common focus on affect, behaviors, and cognitions. For the purpose of this article, the authors simply refer to the entire group of interventions as CBT. Meta-analyses of randomized controlled trials show CBT is effective for anxiety[9–14] and depression.[15,16] Unfortunately, a substantial minority of patients do not respond to CBT. For example, in several studies nonresponse rates for panic disorder, obsessive-compulsive disorder, and social anxiety disorder were 36%, 38%, and 49%, respectively.[17–20] Treatment development guidelines state that improving interventions requires a better understanding of the change process.[21,22] Thus, CBT researchers are seeking to identify core mechanisms of change (treatment mediators) in an effort to develop effective augmentation strategies or new interventions.[23–25]

Mediators are variables that can explain why or how a treatment works, and they are measured at least at pretreatment and posttreatment. Early analysis strategies (**Fig. 1**) suggested mediation if (1) the treatment-affected outcome (path *a*), (2) the mediator-affected outcome (path *b*), and (3) while controlling for the mediator (paths *a* and *b*), the effect of treatment on outcome was reduced or eliminated.[26]

However, with only these limited criteria for mediation, there were many false positives.[27] Over time, several more mediation criteria were proposed.[28,29] A more comprehensive strategy was suggested by Kazdin.[30] In addition to showing statistical mediation, the following 7 additional criteria were recommended: (1) mediators should be selected guided by theory, (2) potential mediators must be measured in treatment studies, (3) temporal precedence must be established (change in the proposed mediator must occur before change in outcome), (4) more than one mediator should be measured in each study to establish specificity, (5) the design of the study should be sufficient to evaluate mediators, (6) multiple different studies must show similar evidence, (7) the mediator should be directly manipulated to provide converging evidence. These criteria add confidence in the causal relationship between the independent variable (treatment), the mediator, and the dependent variable (outcome measures). Many more recent studies meet criteria 1 through 6. However, studies meeting criteria 7 remain limited.[31] These criteria are not without limitations. For example, if mediators need to be theory driven (criteria 1), the strength of the literature depends on the strength of the theory. Thus, if the actual mechanism of change is not theorized or measured, it will remain undetected with this approach. Nevertheless, this approach has been fruitful to date.

Many mediators of CBT have been proposed (eg, self-efficacy,[32] emotional processing theory fear network modification[33]). However, most can be roughly collapsed into either behavioral[34] or cognitive[35] processes. The behavioral perspective began primarily as a method (exposure) that evolved into an explanation (extinction learning) beginning with Dr Joseph Wolpe's work with cats.[34,36–39] The cognitive perspective of Dr Aaron T. Beck and colleagues[35] focused on changes in thinking as an explanation

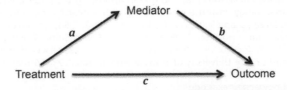

Fig. 1. Baron and Kenny suggested mediation when (1) the treatment affected outcome (*path a*), (2) the mediator affected outcome (*path b*), and (3) while controlling for the mediator (*paths a and b*), the effect of treatment on outcome was reduced or eliminated.

for symptom improvement regardless of the method (eg, cognitive restructuring, behavioral experiments).[40,41] In later discussion, the authors discuss each of these in turn. However, the division of the 2 may be artificial. For example, Hofmann[42] suggested that extinction learning may be cognitively mediated by changes in harm expectancies.

ANXIETY DISORDERS: THE BEHAVIORAL PERSPECTIVE: FEAR EXTINCTION

In this section, the authors discuss the most researched mechanism of change in CBT for anxiety and related disorders.[43] More specifically, they discuss fear extinction as a model for exposure therapy for the treatment of anxiety and related disorders. In this model, anxiety disorders may be acquired via Pavlovian classical conditioning and maintained through operant conditioning (avoidance with negative reinforcement).[44] For example, a soldier may survive a nearby explosion while riding in a Humvee. In this example, the Humvee is the neutral stimulus, the explosion is the unconditioned stimulus (US), and fear is the unconditioned response. This pairing can result in the Humvee becoming a conditioned stimulus (CS) that also causes fear (conditioned response). If the soldier avoids the thoughts, images, and other reminders, this relationship between the Humvee stimulus and fear can persist. One advantage of this model is that it can be tested experimentally in animals and humans. The subject can undergo acquisition (pairing of the CS and aversive US), extinction (repeatedly presenting the CS without the US), and a test phase (presenting the CS again in a different context to test generalization and maintenance of gains). This research led to many important findings on optimal fear extinction parameters[45,46] and reasons for relapse.[38,39]

Although fear extinction is frequently referred to as a mechanism of fear reduction, it is not the final level of analysis. Two major theories on how fear extinction operates include habituation and inhibitory learning.[38,47-50] Habituation refers to the process of automated fear reduction in response to prolonged exposure to a feared stimulus. Although habituation may be operating during extinction, far more research has come from the inhibitory learning literature.[38,51] This theory describes the process of extinction and emerged from findings that exposure therapy does not appear to erase the fear memory, but rather competes with it.[39,52,53] After successful exposure therapy, many patients experience a return of fear. This return suggests that the fear memory was never entirely erased. There are 4 primary categories of return of fear including spontaneous recovery, renewal, reinstatement, and rapid reacquisition.[38,39] Spontaneous recovery is the return of fear that occurs with the passage of time. Renewal is a return of fear that is brought on by a shift in context that is different from the extinction context. Reinstatement can occur when the patient experiences another US that brings back the association between the CS and US. Finally, rapid reacquisition occurs if the CS and US are parried again after extinction (the fear response is learned much faster than if they had never previously been paired). Interestingly, each of these can be addressed by modifying the exposure protocol.[50] The authors discuss a summary of these modifications in later discussion. First, they cover a summary of research on extinction in anxiety disorders.

Research shows that participants with anxiety disorders respond differently during fear acquisition and extinction. Overall, they show greater and more generalized fear responses during acquisition, and they are more resistant to extinction.[6,54,55] Duits and colleagues[55] examined 44 studies in their meta-analysis of classical fear conditioning in the anxiety disorders. Results showed increased fear responses among anxiety patients to conditioned safety cues (CS–) during fear acquisition. Increased responses to safety cues suggest that they may have a tendency to overgeneralize fear learning. In addition, they showed greater fear responses to the CS+ during extinction indicative of reduced or delayed extinction of the fear response. Other studies show that the level of extinction in a pretreatment assessment predicts the level of improvement in CBT for anxiety disorders.[7,56] Lueken and colleagues[7] examined neural correlates of fear conditioning and extinction before and after CBT for panic disorder. They found that altered safety signal processing demonstrates individual differences that determine the effectiveness of CBT. Interestingly, successful CBT also appears to improve extinction parameters in anxiety patients. Posttreatment, anxiety disorder patients show a better response to extinction, possibly associated with increased prefrontal cortex activity and better coupling between the amygdala, insula, and the anterior cingulate cortex.[6–8]

As stated, research on extinction as a mechanism of change produced several augmentation suggestions to improve CBT for anxiety disorders.[50,57] These suggestions include the following: (1) maximize the mismatch between the expected and actual outcome (expectancy violation),[58] (2) fade use of safety behaviors (safety signals),[59] (3) combine multiple fear stimuli (deepened extinction), (4) occasionally pair the fear stimulus with an aversive outcome (occasional reinforcement),[60] (5) vary the stimuli including intertrial intervals (variability),[61] (6) conduct exposure in multiple contexts,[61–63] (7) label the emotional content (affect labeling),[64] (8) sleep after extinction,[65] (9) deliver exposure during sleep,[66] (10) combine the feared stimulus with a neutral stimulus during extinction (novelty outcome),[67] (11) combine feared stimulus with less aversive outcome (US devaluation),[68] (12) use retrieval cues,[69,70] (13) induce positive mood before extinction,[71] (14) engage in physical exercise before extinction,[72,73] (15) expose a novel context before or after extinction,[74–76] (16) activate the fear memory briefly before extinction training (reconsolidation).[77,78] This list is not exhaustive and does not cover pharmacologic enhancement of fear extinction.[79–86] For a recent review of these strategies in OCD, see Jacoby and Abramowitz.[87] However, this research is still emerging. For many of these strategies, there is preclinical evidence that they facilitate or enhance consolidation of extinction learning, but whether these strategies indeed enhance CBT outcome needs further investigation.

ANXIETY DISORDERS: THE COGNITIVE PERSPECTIVE: THREAT REAPPRAISAL MEDIATION HYPOTHESIS

The cognitive perspective can be divided among automatic and conscious cognitive processes. The relationship between the 2 is described as the "horse and rider" metaphor.[88,89] The horse refers to the automatic processes (attention bias, approach bias, interpretive bias, and so forth) and is the subject of cognitive bias modification research. The work in this area is relatively new and shows promising but at times conflicting results.[90–94] Thus, for the purpose of the current article, the authors focus on "the rider." The rider here refers to the more volitional conscious cognitive misappraisal activity that is modified through cognitive or behavioral methods. The 2 most common cognitive errors from this perspective are likelihood and cost overestimations of threat.[40] Patients with anxiety disorders tend to overestimate how likely a negative outcome will be (I will be anxious in every social situation; people will always notice; they will always assume I am incompetent). They also overestimate how bad the outcome will be (cost: if a person thinks I am incompetent, this means all people will think I'm incompetent and I will die alone). These faulty threat appraisals then lead to avoidance or escape that maintains the disorder.[35] CBT seeks to target these faulty threat appraisals through exposure and cognitive restructuring. The overarching goal is threat reappraisal and resulting symptom improvement (reduced anxiety). Thus, threat reappraisal is a proposed mediator for the efficacy of CBT in anxiety disorders.[42]

In an effort to summarize this literature, the authors conducted a systematic review that identified 25 studies that examined the threat reappraisal mediation hypothesis in panic disorder, social anxiety disorder, obsessive-compulsive disorder, posttraumatic stress disorder, acute stress disorder, specific phobia, and one study with a mixed population.[31] The authors included studies that (1) investigated the threat reappraisal mediation hypothesis, (2) included adults with and anxiety disorder, and (3) included a longitudinal design. First, results showed that 56% of the studies investigated statistical mediation, and all but one of those (13 of 14 studies) demonstrated either a significant mediated pathway or a reduction of the strength of the relation between treatment and anxiety reduction after controlling for threat reappraisal. Second, 28% of the studies demonstrated evidence for a causal relation between CBT and threat reappraisal. Third, 28% of the studies examined whether threat reappraisal caused anxiety reduction, and all but one of those (6 of 7 studies) demonstrated that threat reappraisal resulted in subsequent reductions in anxiety. Finally, 44% of the studies controlled for one or more plausible alternative mediators, and 9 of 11 studies observed significant relations between threat reappraisal and anxiety reduction after controlling for one or more plausible alternative mediators. Thus, there was strong evidence of the association between threat reappraisal and symptom reduction. However, there was less evidence that threat reappraisal *caused* symptom reduction - particularly in OCD. [95] For example, Woody and colleagues[95] found evidence of statistical mediation, that CBT caused threat reappraisal, and the effect was specific. However, they also showed that threat reappraisal did not cause anxiety reduction.

Based on this literature, recommendations for CBT for anxiety disorders include enhancing threat reappraisal through several methods. Patients are expected to make their threat predictions explicit (both likelihood and cost estimations). They are then encouraged to attend to and evaluate these predictions during and after exposure trials. Thus, they are guided to attend to their core threats, evaluate them, and then summarize what is learned in an effort to enhance the threat reappraisal.

ANXIETY DISORDERS: CURRENT TRENDS

Until this point, the authors have largely discussed mechanisms of fear reduction. Understandably, patients approach them for exactly this purpose. However, many studies show that not every person has a steady decline in anxiety (either within or across sessions). Nevertheless, this often does not negatively impact long-term success. For example, extinction data show that the amount of fear reduction during extinction training does not always predict the amount of fear at retest.[96–98] Similarly, the amount of fear reduction during exposure therapy does not always predict the amount of fear at follow-up.[99–101] Therefore, the focus on fear as the primary target shifted to a focus on function and adaptive value guided behavior regardless of anxiety or mood. Resulting treatments include mindfulness-based approaches and acceptance and commitment therapy.[102,103] There is debate whether this should be considered a "new wave" of CBT or simply the continued refocus away from immediate anxiety reduction in favor of long-term improved quality of life.[104] Hofmann and colleagues[105] reviewed the literature and suggested that the new approaches are similar in efficacy to CBT and that these new therapies are consistent with the CBT approach.

There is some debate on whether the authors should even measure fear during treatment sessions because this sends a message that it must be dangerous.[87] However, it would difficult to convince a patient that they do not intend to reduce the very symptom they are presenting with for treatment. Rather, one way of presenting this rationale is to say that, at least during the course of treatment, the goal is not to win the war but rather to stop fighting. However, an important follow-up is to state that when one stops fighting during the course of treatment, the war eventually ceases (and the patient has achieved his treatment goals). Similarly, with anxiety, once one no longer finds anxiety threatening, it too eventually goes away. This second part of the message is often neglected in clinical and research settings.

DEPRESSION: COGNITIVE MECHANISMS

Cognitions figure prominently in the research and treatment literature for depression. Not surprisingly, cognitive change is the most researched mediator of CBT for depression. Beck[106] first developed a comprehensive theory of the cause and maintaining factors for major depression. Central to the theory was the role of inaccurate beliefs and maladaptive information processing (repetitive negative thinking). The cognitive model suggests that when these errors in thinking are corrected (cognitive change) that depression lessens and the likelihood of relapse is reduced. Interestingly, early studies suggested both antidepressants and CBT produced similar levels of cognitive change. However, careful follow-up studies and analysis showed that cognitive changes precede symptom improvement in CBT but not in the medication conditions.[107–110] For example, DeRubeis and colleagues[110] randomized outpatients with major depression to CBT or pharmacotherapy and measured cognitions and symptoms at pretreatment, mid treatment, and at posttreatment (week 12). They found that changes from pretreatment to mid treatment on cognitive measures (the Automatic Thoughts Questionnaire, Dysfunctional Attitudes Scale, and the Hopelessness Scale) significantly predicted change in depression from mid treatment to posttreatment. Cognitive change also predicts lower relapse rates.[111–114] Teasdale and colleagues[112] examined how cognitive therapy prevented relapse among 158 patients with residual depression. They found that relapse was reduced by reductions in absolute, dichotomous thinking styles. In an attempt to further determine the specificity of cognitive change, Jacobson and colleagues[115] conducted a dismantling study randomizing patients to behavioral activation alone, behavioral activation plus modification of automatic thoughts, or behavioral activation with modification of both automatic thoughts and schemas. Overall, they found the 3 treatments were equally efficacious. Their data also suggested that cognitive change was important but not differentially affected by the different treatments as one might expect. Thus, cognitive change is important in CBT for depression in whatever manner it is achieved. Finally, research on "sudden gains" in depression further supports the role of cognitive change as a mediator. Sudden gains refers to a relatively sudden drop in depressive symptoms during CBT (an average drop of 11 points on the Beck Depression Inventory that occurs between sessions 4 and 8 in approximately 30%–50% of patients).[116–120] Importantly, Tang and colleagues[116,118] found that cognitive change predicted sudden gains. In 2 studies, they found more cognitive change in the sessions preceding sudden gains relative to other control sessions in the same patients.

SUMMARY

There have been great strides in the development of effective treatments for anxiety and depression. However, a substantial minority of patients do not respond or do not fully recover. Recommendations in the field are to identify mechanisms of change to guide the search for augmentation strategies or the development of future CBT. The most evidence in the anxiety disorders currently is for mediation described by fear extinction and threat reappraisal. Interestingly, these 2 theories are not incompatible and may represent differences in levels of analysis. The same can be said for research on brain mechanisms. Across anxiety and depression, there is agreement that the limbic system and prefrontal cortex are intricately involved in the process of change. The most researched psychological mechanism in CBT for depression is cognitive change. Cognitive change is observed in both antidepressant and CBT interventions. It is also observed in both cognitive (cognitive restructuring) and behavioral (behavioral activation) therapies. Overall, cognitive change is important in CBT for both anxiety and depression in whatever manner it is achieved. It may be that cognitive change is important, and one of the best ways to convince someone to change their mind is through giving them experience (exposure/behavioral experiments). Thus, exposure and behavioral interventions may be very good cognitive therapy.

REFERENCES

1. Smits JA, Hofmann SG. A meta-analytic review of the effects of psychotherapy control conditions for anxiety disorders. Psychol Med 2009;39:229–39.
2. Goldapple K, Segal Z, Garson C, et al. Modulation of cortical-limbic pathways in major depression: treatment-specific effects of cognitive behavior therapy. Arch Gen Psychiatry 2004;61:34–41.
3. Saxena S, Brody AL, Ho ML, et al. Differential cerebral metabolic changes with paroxetine treatment of obsessive-compulsive disorder vs major depression. Arch Gen Psychiatry 2002;59:250–61.
4. Kennedy SH, Evans KR, Krüger S, et al. Changes in regional brain glucose metabolism measured with positron emission tomography after paroxetine treatment of major depression. Am J Psychiatry 2001;158:899–905.
5. Mayberg HS, Brannan SK, Tekell JL, et al. Regional metabolic effects of fluoxetine in major depression: serial changes and relationship to clinical response. Biol Psychiatry 2000;48:830–43.
6. Duits P, Cath DC, Heitland I, et al. High current anxiety symptoms, but not a past anxiety disorder diagnosis, are associated with impaired fear extinction. Front Psychol 2016;7:252.
7. Lueken U, Straube B, Konrad C, et al. Neural substrates of treatment response to cognitive-behavioral therapy in panic disorder with agoraphobia. Am J Psychiatry 2013;170:1345–55.
8. Schienle A, Schäfer A, Hermann A, et al. Symptom provocation and reduction in patients suffering from spider phobia: an fMRI study on exposure therapy. Eur Arch Psychiatry Clin Neurosci 2007;257:486–93.
9. Hofmann SG, Smits JAJ. Cognitive-behavioral therapy for adult anxiety disorders: a meta-analysis of randomized placebo-controlled trials. J Clin Psychiatry 2008;69:621–32.
10. Powers MB, Halpern JM, Ferenschak MP, et al. A meta-analytic review of prolonged exposure for posttraumatic stress disorder. Clin Psychol Rev 2010;30: 635–41.
11. Olatunji BO, Davis ML, Powers MB, et al. Cognitive-behavioral therapy for obsessive-compulsive disorder: a meta-analysis of treatment outcome and moderators. J Psychiatr Res 2013;47:33–41.

12. Wolitzky-Taylor KB, Horowitz JD, Powers MB, et al. Psychological approaches in the treatment of specific phobias: a meta-analysis. Clin Psychol Rev 2008;28: 1021–37.

13. Powers MB, Sigmarsson SR, Emmelkamp PMGA. Meta-analytic review of psychological treatments for social anxiety disorder. Int J Cogn Ther 2008;1: 94–113.

14. Olatunji BO, Kauffman BY, Meltzer S, et al. Cognitive-behavioral therapy for hypochondriasis/health anxiety: a meta-analysis of treatment outcome and moderators. Behav Res Ther 2014;58:65–74.

15. Cuijpers P, Berking M, Andersson G, et al. A meta-analysis of cognitive-behavioural therapy for adult depression, alone and in comparison with other treatments. Can J Psychiatry 2013;58:376–85.

16. Hofmann SG, Asnaani A, Vonk IJJ, et al. The efficacy of cognitive behavioral therapy: a review of meta-analyses. Cogn Ther Res 2012;36:427–40.

17. Barlow DH, Gorman JM, Shear MK, et al. Cognitive-behavioral therapy, imipramine, or their combination for panic disorder: a randomized controlled trial. JAMA 2000;283:2529–36.

18. Borkovec TD, Costello E. Efficacy of applied relaxation and cognitive-behavioral therapy in the treatment of generalized anxiety disorder. J Consult Clin Psychol 1993;61:611–9.

19. Davidson JRT, Foa EB, Huppert JD, et al. Fluoxetine, comprehensive cognitive behavioral therapy, and placebo in generalized social phobia. Arch Gen Psychiatry 2004;61:1005–13.

20. Foa EB, Liebowitz MR, Kozak MJ, et al. Randomized, placebo-controlled trial of exposure and ritual prevention, clomipramine, and their combination in the treatment of obsessive-compulsive disorder. Am J Psychiatry 2005;162:151–61.

21. Kazdin A. Progression of therapy research and clinical application of treatment require better understanding of the change process. Clin Psychooogy Sci Pract 2001;8:143–51.

22. Rounsaville BJ, Carroll KM, Onken LS. A stage model of behavioral therapies research: Getting started and moving from stage 11. Clin Psychol Sci Pract 2001;8:133–42.

23. Hofmann SG. Common misconceptions about cognitive mediation of treatment change: a commentary to Longmore and Worrell (2007). Clin Psychol Rev 2008; 28:67–70.

24. Hofmann SG, Meuret AE, Rosenfield D, et al. Preliminary evidence for cognitive mediation during cognitive-behavioral therapy of panic disorder. J Consult Clin Psychol 2007;75:374–9.

25. Smits JAJ, Powers MB, Cho Y, et al. Mechanism of change in cognitive-behavioral treatment of panic disorder: evidence for the fear of fear mediational hypothesis. J Consult Clin Psychol 2004;72:646–52.

26. Baron RM, Kenny DA. The moderator-mediator variable distinction in social psychological research: conceptual, strategic, and statistical considerations. J Pers Soc Psychol 1986;51:1173–82.

27. Maxwell SE, Cole DA. Bias in cross-sectional analyses of longitudinal mediation. Psychol Methods 2007;12:23–44.

28. Kraemer HC, Wilson GT, Fairburn CG, et al. Mediators and moderators of treatment effects in randomized clinical trials. Arch Gen Psychiatry 2002;59:877–83.

29. Kraemer HC, Kiernan M, Essex M, et al. How and why criteria defining moderators and mediators differ between the Baron & Kenny and MacArthur approaches. Health Psychol 2008;27:S101–8.

30. Kazdin AE. Mediators and mechanisms of change in psychotherapy research. Annu Rev Clin Psychol 2007;3:1–27.

31. Smits JAJ, Julian K, Rosenfield D, et al. Threat reappraisal as a mediator of symptom change in cognitive-behavioral treatment of anxiety disorders: a systematic review. J Consult Clin Psychol 2012;80:624–35.

32. Bandura A. Self-efficacy: toward a unifying theory of behavioral change. Psychol Rev 1977;84:191–215.

33. Foa EB, Kozak MJ. Emotional processing of fear: exposure to corrective information. Psychol Bull 1986;99:20–35.

34. Wolpe J. Psychotherapy by reciprocal inhibition. Redwood City (CA): Stanford University Press; 1958.

35. Beck AT, Emery G, Greenberg RL. Anxiety disorders and phobias: a cognitive perspective. New York: Basic Books; 1985.

36. Quirk GJ. Memory for extinction of conditioned fear is long-lasting and persists following spontaneous recovery. Learn Mem 2002;9:402–7.

37. Kindt M. A behavioural neuroscience perspective on the aetiology and treatment of anxiety disorders. Behav Res Ther 2014;62:24–36.

38. Bouton ME. Context, time, and memory retrieval in the interference paradigms of Pavlovian learning. Psychol Bull 1993;114:80–99.

39. Bouton ME. Context, ambiguity, and unlearning: sources of relapse after behavioral extinction. Biol Psychiatry 2002;52:976–86.

40. Clark DA, Beck AT. Cognitive theory and therapy of anxiety and depression: convergence with neurobiological findings. Trends Cogn Sci 2010;14:418–24.

41. Hollon SD, Stewart MO, Strunk D. Enduring effects for cognitive behavior therapy in the treatment of depression and anxiety. Annu Rev Psychol 2006;57: 285–315.

42. Hofmann SG. Cognitive processes during fear acquisition and extinction in animals and humans: implications for exposure therapy of anxiety disorders. Clin Psychol Rev 2008;28:199–210.

43. Kazdin AE. Understanding how and why psychotherapy leads to change. Psychother Res 2009;19:418–28.

44. Mowrer OH. Learning theory and behavior. New York: Wiley; 1960.

45. Cain CK, Blouin AM, Barad M. Temporally massed CS presentations generate more fear extinction than spaced presentations. J Exp Psychol Anim Behav Process 2003;29:323–33.

46. Rescorla RA. Extinction can be enhanced by a concurrent excitor. J Exp Psychol Anim Behav Process 2000;26:251–60.

47. Rachman S, Levitt K. Panic, fear reduction and habituation. Behav Res Ther 1988;26:199–206.

48. Lader MH, Mathews AM. A physiological model of phobic anxiety and desensitization. Behav Res Ther 1968;6:411–21.

49. Watts FN. Habituation model of systematic desensitization. Psychol Bull 1979; 86:627–37.

50. Craske MG, Treanor M, Conway C, et al. Maximizing exposure therapy: an inhibitory learning approach. Behav Res Ther 2014;58:10–23.

51. Myers KM, Davis M. Mechanisms of fear extinction. Mol Psychiatry 2007;12: 120–50.

52. Eisenberg M, Kobilo T, Berman DE, et al. Stability of retrieved memory: inverse correlation with trace dominance. Science 2003;301:1102–4.

53. Alfei JM, Ferrer Monti RI, Molina VA, et al. Prediction error and trace dominance determine the fate of fear memories after post-training manipulations. Learn Mem 2015;22:385–400.

54. Lissek S, Powers AS, McClure EB, et al. Classical fear conditioning in the anxiety disorders: a meta-analysis. Behav Res Ther 2005;43:1391–424.

55. Duits P, Cath DC, Lissek S, et al. Updated meta-analysis of classical fear conditioning in the anxiety disorders. Depress Anxiety 2015;32:239–53.

56. Hahn T, Kircher T, Straube B, et al. Predicting treatment response to cognitive behavioral therapy in panic disorder with agoraphobia by integrating local neural information. JAMA Psychiatry 2015;72:68–74.

57. Pittig A, van den Berg L, Vervliet B. The key role of extinction learning in anxiety disorders: behavioral strategies to enhance exposure-based treatments. Curr Opin Psychiatry 2015;28:1–9.

58. Deacon B, Kemp JJ, Dixon LJ, et al. Maximizing the efficacy of interoceptive exposure by optimizing inhibitory learning: a randomized controlled trial. Behav Res Ther 2013;51:588–96.

59. Powers MB, Smits JAJ, Telch MJ. Disentangling the effects of safety-behavior utilization and safety-behavior availability during exposure-based treatment: a placebo-controlled trial. J Consult Clin Psychol 2004;72:448–54.

60. Culver N. Extinction-based processes for enhancing the effectiveness of exposure therapy. Los Angeles (CA): eScholarship; 2013.

61. Shiban Y, Schelhorn I, Pauli P, et al. Effect of combined multiple contexts and multiple stimuli exposure in spider phobia: a randomized clinical trial in virtual reality. Behav Res Ther 2015;71:45–53.

62. Bandarian-Balooch S, Neumann DL, Boschen MJ. Exposure treatment in multiple contexts attenuates return of fear via renewal in high spider fearful individuals. J Behav Ther Exp Psychiatry 2015;47:138–44.

63. Dunsmoor JE, Ahs F, Zielinski DJ, et al. Extinction in multiple virtual reality contexts diminishes fear reinstatement in humans. Neurobiol Learn Mem 2014;113: 157–64.

64. Niles AN, Craske MG, Lieberman MD, et al. Affect labeling enhances exposure effectiveness for public speaking anxiety. Behav Res Ther 2015;68:27–36.

65. Kleim B, Wilhelm FH, Temp L, et al. Sleep enhances exposure therapy. Psychol Med 2014;44:1511–9.

66. He J, Sun HQ, Li SX, et al. Effect of conditioned stimulus exposure during slow wave sleep on fear memory extinction in humans. Sleep 2015;38:423–31.

67. Dunsmoor JE, Campese VD, Ceceli AO, et al. Novelty-facilitated extinction: providing a novel outcome in place of an expected threat diminishes recovery of defensive responses. Biol Psychiatry 2015;78:203–9.

68. Haesen K, Vervliet B. Beyond extinction: habituation eliminates conditioned skin conductance across contexts. Int J Psychophysiol 2015;98:529–34.

69. Culver NC, Stoyanova M, Craske MG. Clinical relevance of retrieval cues for attenuating context renewal of fear. J Anxiety Disord 2011;25:284–92.

70. Mystkowski JL, Craske MG, Echiverri AM, et al. Mental reinstatement of context and return of fear in spider-fearful participants. Behav Ther 2006;37:49–60.

71. Zbozinek TD, Holmes EA, Craske MG. The effect of positive mood induction on reducing reinstatement fear: relevance for long term outcomes of exposure therapy. Behav Res Ther 2015;71:65–75.

72. Powers MB, Medina JL, Burns S, et al. Exercise augmentation of exposure therapy for PTSD: rationale and pilot efficacy data. Cogn Behav Ther 2015;44: 314–27.

73. Siette J, Reichelt AC, Westbrook RF. A bout of voluntary running enhances context conditioned fear, its extinction, and its reconsolidation. Learn Mem 2014;21:73–81.

74. de Carvalho Myskiw J, Benetti F, Izquierdo I. Behavioral tagging of extinction learning. Proc Natl Acad Sci U S A 2013;110:1071–6.

75. Menezes J, Alves N, Borges S, et al. Facilitation of fear extinction by novelty depends on dopamine acting on D1-subtype dopamine receptors in hippocampus. Proc Natl Acad Sci U S A 2015;112:E1652–8.

76. de Carvalho Myskiw J, Furini CRG, Benetti F, et al. Hippocampal molecular mechanisms involved in the enhancement of fear extinction caused by exposure to novelty. Proc Natl Acad Sci U S A 2014;111:4572–7.

77. Schiller D, Monfils MH, Raio CM, et al. Preventing the return of fear in humans using reconsolidation update mechanisms. Nature 2010;463:49–53.

78. Soeter M, Kindt M. Dissociating response systems: erasing fear from memory. Neurobiol Learn Mem 2010;94:30–41.

79. Smits JAJ, Monfils MH, Raio CM, et al. D-cycloserine enhancement of fear extinction is specific to successful exposure sessions: evidence from the treatment of height phobia. Biol Psychiatry 2013;73:1054–8.

80. Meyerbroeker K, Powers MB, van Stegeren A, et al. Does yohimbine hydrochloride facilitate fear extinction in virtual reality treatment of fear of flying? A randomized placebo-controlled trial. Psychother Psychosom 2012;81:29–37.

81. Powers MB, Smits JAJ, Otto MW, et al. Facilitation of fear extinction in phobic participants with a novel cognitive enhancer: a randomized placebo controlled trial of yohimbine augmentation. J Anxiety Disord 2009;23:350–6.

82. Smits JAJ, Rosenfield D, Davis ML, et al. Yohimbine enhancement of exposure therapy for social anxiety disorder: a randomized controlled trial. Biol Psychiatry 2014;75:840–6.

83. Hofmann SG. D-cycloserine for treating anxiety disorders: making good exposures better and bad exposures worse. Depress Anxiety 2014;31:175–7.

84. Tart CD, Handelsman PR, Deboer LB, et al. Augmentation of exposure therapy with post-session administration of D-cycloserine. J Psychiatr Res 2013;47:168–74.

85. Hofmann SG, Otto MW, Pollack MH, et al. D-cycloserine augmentation of cognitive behavioral therapy for anxiety disorders: an update. Curr Psychiatry Rep 2015;17:532.

86. Hofmann SG, Smits JA, Rosenfield D, et al. D-cycloserine as an augmentation strategy with cognitive-behavioral therapy for social anxiety disorder. Am J Psychiatry 2013;170:751–8.

87. Jacoby RJ, Abramowitz JS. Inhibitory learning approaches to exposure therapy: a critical review and translation to obsessive-compulsive disorder. Clin Psychol Rev 2016;49:28–40.

88. Wiers RW, Gladwin TE, Hofmann W, et al. Cognitive bias modification and cognitive control training in addiction and related psychopathology: mechanisms, clinical perspectives, and ways forward. Clin Psychol Sci 2013;1:192–212.

89. Friese M, Hofmann W, Wiers RW. On taming horses and strengthening riders: recent developments in research on interventions to improve self-control in health behaviors. Self Identity 2011;10:336–51.

90. Julian K, Beard C, Schmidt NB, et al. Attention training to reduce attention bias and social stressor reactivity: an attempt to replicate and extend previous findings. Behav Res Ther 2012;50:350–8.

91. Baird SO, Rinck M, Rosenfield D, et al. Reducing approach bias to achieve smoking cessation: a pilot randomized placebo-controlled trial. Cogn Ther Res 2017;1–9. http://dx.doi.org/10.1007/s10608-017-9835-z.

92. Cristea IA, Kok RN, Cuijpers P. Efficacy of cognitive bias modification interventions in anxiety and depression: meta-analysis. Br J Psychiatry 2015;206:7–16.

93. Linetzky M, Pergamin-Hight L, Pine DS, et al. Quantitative evaluation of the clinical efficacy of attention bias modification treatment for anxiety disorders. Depress Anxiety 2015;32:383–91.

94. MacLeod C, Grafton B. Anxiety-linked attentional bias and its modification: illustrating the importance of distinguishing processes and procedures in experimental psychopathology research. Behav Res Ther 2016;86:68–86.

95. Woody SR, Whittal ML, McLean PD. Mechanisms of symptom reduction in treatment for obsessions. J Consult Clin Psychol 2011;79:653–64.

96. Plendl W, Wotjak CT. Dissociation of within- and between-session extinction of conditioned fear. J Neurosci 2010;30:4990–8.

97. Prenoveau JM, Craske MG, Liao B, et al. Human fear conditioning and extinction: timing is everything... or is it? Biol Psychol 2013;92:59–68.

98. Rescorla RA. Deepened extinction from compound stimulus presentation. J Exp Psychol 2006;32:135–44.

99. Baker A, Mystkowski J, Culver N, et al. Does habituation matter? Emotional processing theory and exposure therapy for acrophobia. Behav Res Ther 2010;48:1139–43.

100. Culver NC, Stoyanova M, Craske MG. Emotional variability and sustained arousal during exposure. J Behav Ther Exp Psychiatry 2012;43:787–93.

101. Kircanski K, Mortazavi A, Castriotta N, et al. Challenges to the traditional exposure paradigm: variability in exposure therapy for contamination fears. J Behav Ther Exp Psychiatry 2012;43:745–51.

102. Powers MB, Zum Vorde Sive Vording MB, Emmelkamp PMG. Acceptance and commitment therapy: a meta-analytic review. Psychother Psychosom 2009;78:73–80.

103. A-Tjak JG, Davis ML, Morina N, et al. A meta-analysis of the efficacy of acceptance and commitment therapy for clinically relevant mental and physical health problems. Psychother Psychosom 2015;84:30–6.

104. Hofmann SG, Asmundson GJG. Acceptance and mindfulness-based therapy: new wave or old hat? Clin Psychol Rev 2008;28:1–16.

105. Hofmann SG, Sawyer AT, Fang A. The empirical status of the 'new wave' of CBT. Psychiatr Clin North Am 2010;33:701–10.

106. Beck AT. Cognitive therapy of depression. New York: Guilford Press; 1979.

107. Imber SD, Pilkonis PA, Sotsky SM, et al. Mode-specific effects among three treatments for depression. J Consult Clin Psychol 1990;58:352–9.

108. Simons AD, Garfield SL, Murphy GE. The process of change in cognitive therapy and pharmacotherapy for depression. Changes in mood and cognition. Arch Gen Psychiatry 1984;41:45–51.

109. Hollon SD, DeRubeis RJ, Evans MD. Causal mediation of change in treatment for depression: discriminating between nonspecificity and noncausality. Psychol Bull 1987;102:139–49.

110. DeRubeis RJ, Evans MD, Hollon SD, et al. How does cognitive therapy work? Cognitive change and symptom change in cognitive therapy and pharmacotherapy for depression. J Consult Clin Psychol 1990;58:862–9.

111. Strunk DR, DeRubeis RJ, Chiu AW, et al. Patients' competence in and performance of cognitive therapy skills: relation to the reduction of relapse risk following treatment for depression. J Consult Clin Psychol 2007;75:523–30.
112. Teasdale JD, Scott J, Moore RG, et al. How does cognitive therapy prevent relapse in residual depression? Evidence from a controlled trial. J Consult Clin Psychol 2001;69:347–57.
113. Beevers CG, Miller IW. Unlinking negative cognition and symptoms of depression: evidence of a specific treatment effect for cognitive therapy. J Consult Clin Psychol 2005;73:68–77.
114. Segal ZV, Kennedy S, Gemar M, et al. Cognitive reactivity to sad mood provocation and the prediction of depressive relapse. Arch Gen Psychiatry 2006; 63:749–55.
115. Jacobson NS, Dobson KS, Truax PA, et al. A component analysis of cognitive-behavioral treatment for depression. J Consult Clin Psychol 1996;64:295–304.
116. Tang TZ, DeRubeis RJ. Sudden gains and critical sessions in cognitive-behavioral therapy for depression. J Consult Clin Psychol 1999;67:894–904.
117. Hardy GE, Cahill J, Stiles WB, et al. Sudden gains in cognitive therapy for depression: a replication and extension. J Consult Clin Psychol 2005;73:59–67.
118. Tang TZ, DeRubeis RJ, Beberman R, et al. Cognitive changes, critical sessions, and sudden gains in cognitive-behavioral therapy for depression. J Consult Clin Psychol 2005;73:168–72.
119. Tang TZ, Derubeis RJ, Hollon SD, et al. Sudden gains in cognitive therapy of depression and depression relapse/recurrence. J Consult Clin Psychol 2007; 75:404–8.
120. Vittengl JR, Clark LA, Jarrett RB. Validity of sudden gains in acute phase treatment of depression. J Consult Clin Psychol 2005;73:173–82.

Homework in Cognitive Behavioral Therapy

A Systematic Review of Adherence Assessment in Anxiety and Depression (2011–2016)

Nikolaos Kazantzis, BA(Hons), MA, PGDipClinPsych, PhD*,
Nicole R. Brownfield, BSc (Hons), Livia Mosely, BEng, BA, PDM,
Alexsandra S. Usatoff, BSc, GDipPsych, GDipProfPsych,
Andrew J. Flighty, BPsychSc

KEYWORDS

- Cognitive behavior therapy • Homework • Adherence • Anxiety • Depression
- Review

KEY POINTS

- Significant attention has been directed toward adherence with CBT homework for anxiety and depressive disorders, and adherence assessment methods have diversified.
- There remains a large component of the adherence process not assessed, with patient effort, engagement, and the known role for treatment appraisals and beliefs necessitating the pursuit of improved adherence assessment methods.
- In CBT, the homework intervention varies across sessions and patients, and tailored assessments that consider both the in-session procedures in discussing the homework, and the patient feedback on its benefits are important for understanding adherence.

Although cognitive behavioral therapy (CBT) has demonstrated efficacy as a therapy for acute phase depression and anxiety disorders,[1–4] as with any psychological intervention, it only works when a patient actually adheres to the treatment recommendations and completes treatment.[5,6] In research studies of CBT, there is increasing concern that adherence with psychological therapies are misunderstood and inaccurately measured.[7–11]

CBT requires significant behavior, cognitive, and lifestyle changes that are often difficult for patients to implement. For example, the behavioral activation component of CBT for depression typically requires patients to keep a diary of their emotions and

Disclosures: See last page of the article.
Cognitive Behavior Therapy Research Unit, Level 4, 18 Innovation Walk, School of Psychological Sciences and Monash Institute of Cognitive and Clinical Neurosciences, Monash University, Melbourne 3800, Australia
* Corresponding author.
E-mail address: Nikolaos.Kazantzis@monash.edu

Psychiatr Clin N Am 40 (2017) 625–639
http://dx.doi.org/10.1016/j.psc.2017.08.001
0193-953X/17/© 2017 Elsevier Inc. All rights reserved.

rate the impact of scheduling more activities than typical. Keeping a diary builds emotional awareness, because it requires increased attention to undesirable mood states, making adherence increasingly difficult over the first few weeks (ie, with a focus on sadness, guilt, annoyance, it is harder to stay motivated and engage in activities designed to lift mood). Cognitive restructuring requires a patient to keep a written log of distressing thoughts when low mood occurs, something many loathe doing shortly after a distressing event.

Although these difficulties are typically overcome in tightly controlled trials, because of added support provided by the study and the typically homogeneous sample, they pose a challenge for the practicing clinician without those added resources and restrictions on patient load.[12]

The related issue of treatment attrition also dilutes the benefits of CBT, especially in clinical settings, where dropout rates are as high as 26%.[6] A recent study on nationwide dissemination of CBT in England reported that 48% of patients dropped out during therapy.[13] Taken together, these studies suggest a substantial portion of patients are not receiving the full benefit of CBT, and there is a need for further research on treatment adherence in this context.

HOMEWORK ADHERENCE EFFECTS

The necessity and potential for negative impact of asking patients to complete therapeutic strategies in order to receive the full treatment effect of CBT have been noted.[14] This view is, in part, due to the terminology used to refer to this practice: "homework" clearly stems from the educational model and to refer to "homework assignments" in therapy does not immediately convey the necessarily collaborative nature of this therapeutic process. Furthermore, although various terminologies have been used in treatment studies, the term "homework" is most consistently used and may be defined as "planned activities the patient carries out between sessions, selected together with the therapist, in order to progress toward therapy goals."[15]

It is not surprising that even modest improvements in homework adherence can enhance CBT outcomes. Findings from 2 independent meta-analyses spanning 1980 to 1998[16] and 2000 to 2008[17] of 1702 and 2183 patients, respectively, found that those with anxiety and depression who completed treatment with higher levels of adherence improved significantly more than completers with low adherence (effect size $r = .22$ for depression, and $r = .24$ for anxiety[16]; and overall $r = .26$[17]). In addition, adherence with treatment strategies is a strong predictor of long-term (ie, 1 year) outcomes.[16] A later meta-analysis of studies spanning 1980 to 2007 of 1072 patients in CBT conditions with and without homework reported that effect sizes for CBT with homework were significantly greater than CBT comprising entirely of in-session work for anxiety and depression ($d = 0.48$).[18]

Conversely, a study by Burns and Spangler[19] observed that there was evidence of a bidirectional relationship between homework adherence and symptom change in CBT for depression.[20] Because the observation of sudden gains has recently been replicated in CBT for depression, the importance of understanding the trajectories of symptom change in CBT cannot be understated.[21] It is possible that homework adherence has a central role in determining sudden symptomatic changes, and therefore, future hypothesis testing to explore the homework adherence-outcome relationship is indicated. The consistent finding that greater homework compliance is associated with positive therapeutic outcomes in interventions for anxiety and depression is itself evidence that homework compliance assessment is important for CBT.

SKILL ACQUISITION: A BROADER CONTEXT FOR ADHERENCE

Unlike pharmacologic interventions, where consistency in treatment protocol is expected, homework may vary considerably in terms of its nature and therapeutic purpose.[22] Even those patients who practice a therapeutic activity, as planned with their therapist, may not receive the clinical benefit, because they may not fully understand the clinical importance of the task. They may adhere out of a desire for approval or acceptance, or indeed, out of a fear of failure, which may also be central to the cause and maintenance of their anxiety or mood disorder.[23] In other instances, patients may invest too much time and effort in their homework, and it may become a source of perceived criticism or rejection. Further still, it is possible that some patients may vary the homework from what was discussed with their therapist, in a manner that may prove more beneficial. CBT homework clearly presents a complex assessment problem.

Ideally, treatment programs would capture not only adherence or compliance with therapeutic homework between sessions (ie, homework "quantity") but also the extent to which the therapeutic homework had been carried out in a skillful and clinically meaningful way (ie, homework "quality").[24,25] Moreover, omitting assessment of therapeutic work between sessions may compromise the utility of wait-list and other comparison group conditions, because patients may elect to engage in self-help or skill practice without clinician prompting.[8]

Patient acquisition of CBT skills arising from treatment adherence can alleviate depression (eg, learning how to manage distressing emotions through increasing pleasant activities, developing skill in testing moment-to-moment negative thoughts, both facilitate reduced symptoms) and anxiety (eg, identify patterns of emotional avoidance; increase awareness and tolerance of emotion-related physical sensations). A recent meta-analysis of studies published from 2008 to 2015 of behavior and cognitive-behavioral therapies for 2312 patients found evidence for comparable adherence-outcome relations, whether homework was assessed based on quantity or quality/skill of completion.[11] Although specific assessment tools have been developed for assessing patient behavioral and cognitive skills, it remains unclear whether such measures are adopted in treatment studies. However, a recent review of methods has not been undertaken.

SYSTEMATIC REVIEW METHODOLOGY

Articles of anxiety and depression published over a 5-year period between 2011 and 2016 were identified through an automated text search of the Embase (via Ovid), PsycINFO (via Ovid), and PubMed databases and required to mention: (a) compliance, or (b) engagement, or (c) adherence, along with at least one of the terms describing homework (**Box 1**). All searches were restricted to human, English, and journal articles to eliminate some of the irrelevant articles. A total of 35,649 potential articles were identified for the review.

MAIN ANALYSES

All Embase, PubMed, and PsycINFO database articles with a title and abstract that met specific predetermined criteria to be more important for homework adherence in psychotherapy were examined: according the following criteria: (a) studies of therapeutic homework in an empirical study of the efficacy of psychotherapy, adopting randomized controlled trial, quasi-experimental, or single-group correlational design; and (b) studies described the assessment of homework quantity or quality within the treatment protocol. With respect to (a), studies that included homework as a component or as the sole basis for treatment (eg, bibliotherapy with a homework component; home-based

---

Box 1
Homework terms used in the systematic review

Activity schedul*

Behavioral experiment*

Behavioral practic*

Behavioural experiment*

Behavioural practic*

Between session

Bibliotherapy

Biofeedback

Exposure

Extra therap*

Extra treatment

Home practice

Homework

Monitoring

Relaxation

Self-help assignment*

Thought record

---

psychological therapy in the treatment of obesity) were included. Studies were excluded if they: (a) focused on specific techniques and not complete therapies (eg, stress reduction) rather than psychotherapies; (b) did not assess treatment outcome (eg, studies of measure validation were excluded); (c) were studies of nonclinical samples; or (d) did not focus on anxiety or depressive disorders. Similarly, studies that (e) measured session attendance or attrition or (f) therapist adherence in order to determine protocol fidelity, without homework adherence assessment, were excluded.

IN-DEPTH MANUAL ASSESSMENT OF HOMEWORK ADHERENCE ASSESSMENT

Article content was first screened to eliminate duplicates using the computer program EndNote (Thomson Reuters EndNote X7, 2013). A total of 14,564 duplicates were identified, resulting in a sample of 20,048 articles to be further screened manually and evaluated for inclusion and exclusion criteria (outlined above) by 3 reviewers (N.B., L.M., and A.U.). Persisting discrepancies were resolved through discussion with a fourth reviewer (N.K.). Data is analyzed independently by a fifth reviewer (A.F.) and cross-checked (N.K.).

RESULTS

A wide variety of measures were used to assess homework adherence in articles published from 2011 to 2016. Among 41 studies of anxiety treatment, 32 (78%) had corresponding details of their assessment methods (**Table 1**).

Overall, 9 studies (22%) included measures assessing the quantity of homework adherence (eg, clinician assessment) based on patient self-report and involved global evaluations (eg, missed none; missed few; missed half, or missed most) or clinician

Table 1
Assessments of homework adherence in studies of psychotherapy for anxiety (2011–2016)

Study	Treatment Model	Homework Adherence Assessment
Alex Brake et al,[37] 2016	CBT for mixed anxiety disorders (N = 7)	The REQ[28] assessed the extent to which participants used different emotion regulation strategies during emotion-eliciting tasks. Participants rated their degree of strategy use from 0 (not at all) to 10 (all the time). A composite score of a combination of mindfulness and avoidance items served as a manipulation check for adherence to instructions.
Anand et al,[38] 2011	CBT for OCD (N = 31)	The single-item HCS[27] was administered at the last therapy session.
Andersson et al,[39] 2011	CBT for OCD (N = 23)	The average number of completed modules from a self-help manual was recorded. Participants submitted homework on completion.
Aviram & Westra,[40] 2011	CBT with or without MI (N = 35)	Therapists rated the degree of client homework compliance throughout CBT using the single-item HCS.[27]
Bluett et al,[41] 2014	Exposure for PTSD (N = 116)	At the beginning of each session, homework adherence was ascertained using the Utility of Techniques Inventory (Foa EB, Hembree EA, Dancu CV. Prolonged exposure (PE) manual: revised version. Unpublished data, 2002), a retrospective self-report measure of both frequency of completion and perceived helpfulness of homework assignments.
Brown et al,[42] 2014	Psychoeducation plus monitoring for PTSD (N = 137)	Participant's monitoring forms were deemed complete if they had recorded at least one numerical frequency rating (of daily reexperiencing of symptoms), and at least one written description of a reexperiencing event from that day, if applicable.
Cammin-Nowak et al,[43] 2013	CBT for panic disorder and agoraphobia (N = 292)	Participants rated the degree to which they completed the homework assigned in the last session on a 7-point Likert scale ranging from 0 (not at all) to 6 (completely done). Quantity of homework completion was also rated by therapists (0 = not at all, 1 = less than assigned, 2 = as assigned, or 3 = more than assigned). Homework quality was rated by the therapist as a global judgment (0 = unsatisfactory, 1 = satisfactory, 2 = good, or 3 = excellent).
Chavira et al,[44] 2014	CBT for mixed anxiety disorders (N = 1004)	Homework adherence was measured as the quantity of homework completed (missed none; missed few; missed half; or missed most).
Cooper et al,[45] 2016	Exposure for PTSD (N = 116)	On the basis of the number of times practiced since the last session, patients rated both in vivo and imaginal homework adherence on a frequency scale from 1 (not at all) to 5 (more than 10 times).

(continued on next page)

Table 1
(continued)

Study	Treatment Model	Homework Adherence Assessment
Dear et al,[46] 2011	CBT for mixed anxiety and depression (N = 32)	The number of participants that completed the 5 lessons within the 8 wk of the program was recorded.
De Kleine et al,[47] 2012	Exposure therapy for PTSD (N = 67)	Homework compliance was measured as the mean number of times per week participants listened to an audiotaped recording of exposure between the sessions.
Dowling et al,[48] 2016	Exposure + response prevention for OCD (N = 49)	The PEAS.[26] Homework adherence was assessed every Monday, Wednesday, and Friday throughout the course of the treatment by a single rater (clinician).
Gershkovich et al,[49] 2016	Internet self-help + ACT/ behavior therapy	Adherence and completion of online modules were monitored each week using software. In addition, the therapist would check if the weekly module was complete before the weekly checkin.
Glenn et al,[50] 2013	CBT for mixed anxiety disorders in primary care (N = 1004)	Two engagement variables: (a) Clinician rating of patient's "overall commitment to CBT this session," rated after every CBT session on a 0- to 10-point scale (0 = *none*, 10 = *complete*); (b) Clinician rating of homework adherence, rated after every CBT session on a 4-point scale (1 = *missed most*, 2 = *missed half*, 3 = *missed few*, and 4 = *missed none*).
Gloster et al,[51] 2011	CBT for panic disorder with agoraphobia (N = 369)	Therapist-rated quality of completed homework was assessed across treatment conditions.
Hundt et al,[52] 2014	CBT for GAD (N = 160)	In each session, the therapist noted the number of homework worksheets completed by each participant. An "average homework completion" variable was created, which measured the total number of worksheets completed divided by the number of treatment sessions completed.
King et al,[53] 2013	MBCT for PTSD (N = 37)	Number of MBCT homework sheets completed, number of minutes listening to audio-recordings on average per d/wk, and number of self-reported time completing informal mindfulness practice throughout the day were recorded.
Lebeau et al,[54] 2013	CBT or ACT for anxiety disorders (N = 84)	The clinician used completed homework log to gauge the proportion of the tasks assigned during the previous session that were completed by the participant during the past week. Ratings were on a scale of 0 (*none completed*) to 4 (*fully completed*). Average of homework compliance ratings across all sessions was calculated.

(continued on next page)

Table 1 *(continued)*		
Study	**Treatment Model**	**Homework Adherence Assessment**
Lewin et al,[55] 2011	CBT for OCD (*N* = 49)	Homework compliance was assessed weekly using a therapist Likert-scale rating (*none, some, moderate, good*). Ratings were informed by parent and child's report of the degree to which homework was completed correctly.
Mataix-Cols et al,[56] 2014	CBT for OCD (*N* = 27)	The PEAS[26]
Meuret et al,[57] 2012	ACT + exposure for panic w/o agoraphobia (*N* = 11)	Homework compliance to ACT exercises (out of 13 per week), assessed via electronic time/date stamp.
Milrod et al,[58] 2016	CBT vs psychodynamic therapy for panic w/o agoraphobia (*N* = 201)	Session-specific, including 3–9 items rated on 1–7 Likert-type scales
Olatunji et al,[59] 2015	CBT for OCD (*N* = 27)	The PEAS[26]
Park et al,[60] 2014	CBT for OCD (*N* = 30)	Therapists assessed quantity and quality of homework compliance weekly at sessions 2–10. Homework compliance ratings were based on parent and child's report of the degree to which the assigned task was completed. The therapist asked general prompts (ie, how did your homework go this week?) at the beginning of each session and could ask follow-up questions, if necessary. Ratings were based on (a) difficulty of exposures completed, (b) amount of habituation experienced during the exposure, (c) deliberateness of the exposure, and (d) the clinician's judgment. This culminated in a rating on a 7-point Likert scale ranging from 0 (*"did not complete any assigned homework"*) to 6 (*"completed all homework and made efforts above and beyond assignments"*).
Ready et al,[61] 2012	Exposure for PTSD (*N* = 30)	The number of times participants reported listening to the recordings of their war-trauma presentations between sessions was recorded.
Robinson et al,[62] 2013	CBT self-help for OCD (*N* = 8)	Participants received weekly telephone calls, which granted an opportunity to assess adherence. Adherence to the intervention was self-reported as the number of chapters they had read of the book.
Simpson et al,[63] 2011	Exposure and response prevention for OCD (*N* = 30)	The PEAS[26]
Westra,[64] 2011	CBT for GAD (*N* = 38)	The single-item Homework Compliance Scale (HCS[27])

(continued on next page)

Table 1 (continued)		
Study	Treatment Model	Homework Adherence Assessment
Wetherell et al,[65] 2016	Exposure for phobia (N = 10)	Number of homework assignments completed
Wheaton et al,[66] 2016	ERP for OCD (N = 37)	The PEAS[26]
Zargar et al,[67] 2013	Acceptance-based behavior therapy vs relaxation for GAD (N = 18)	Engagement in valued actions as measured by the Valued Living Questionnaire.[68]
Zou et al,[69] 2012	CBT (via Internet) for GAD (N = 22)	Percentage of the 5 online lessons completed

Abbreviations: ACT, acceptance and commitment therapy; ERP, exposure and response prevention; GAD, generalized anxiety disorder; HCS, Homework Compliance Scale; MBCT, mindfulness-based cognitive therapy; OCD, obsessive compulsive disorder; PTSD, posttraumatic stress disorder; REQ, Responses to Emotions Questionnaire; w/o, without.

ratings on a Likert scale (eg, 7-point Likert scale ranging from 0 "*did not complete any assigned homework*" to 6 "*completed all homework and made efforts above and beyond assignments*"), and only 3 (7%) involved assessments based completed worksheets, forms, or logs.

Only 2 measures were used consistently across studies: the Patient Adherence to Exposure and Response Prevention Scale (PEAS)[26] was used in 7 studies (17%); and the single-item Homework Compliance Scale[27] was used in 4 studies (10%). The advantage of the PEAS is that it comprises 3 global ratings of quantity (percent of exposures), quality (7-point Likert scale ranging from 1 "*refused*" to 7 "*excellent*"), and response prevention (percent of urges resisted).

Those 6 studies (15%) delivering treatment via technology (eg, Internet) also focused on quantity of completion (ie, modules completed). Only 1 study assessed emotion regulation strategies during tasks (ie, Responses to Emotions Questionnaire),[28] and 1 study sought to corroborate clinician assessment with patient adherence data.

Among 25 studies of depression treatment, only 8 (32%) had corresponding details of their assessment methods (**Table 2**). Overall, 5 studies (20%) included measures to assess the quantity of homework adherence (eg, clinician assessment) based on patient self-report and involved global evaluations (eg, missed none; missed few; missed half, or missed most) or clinician ratings on a Likert scale (eg, 7-point Likert scale ranging from 0 "*no effort*" to 6 "*did more than expected, exceptional effort*"), which assessed engagement (ie, considered effort, obstacles, or difficulty involved in the homework).

Quality of homework completion was assessed in 2 studies (8%): the Mindfulness Homework Practice Questionnaire[29]; and the Homework Rating Scale-Revised,[30] which also assessed theoretically meaningful determinants of adherence. The single study that delivered treatment via technology (eg, Internet) also focused on quantity of completion (ie, modules completed).

DISCUSSION

This evaluation of anxiety and depression studies in the Embase, PsycINFO, and PubMed databases from 2011 to 2016 identified a large number of studies

Table 2
Assessments of homework adherence in studies of psychotherapy for depression (2011–2016)

Study	Treatment Model	Homework Adherence Assessment
Conklin & Strunk,[70] 2015	CT for depression ($N = 53$)	The Homework Engagement Scale—General and Homework Engagement Scale—CT-Specific[70]
Folke et al,[71] 2015	BA for depression ($N = 13$)	In each session the clinician recorded the number and types of assignments from the previous session (eg, activity monitoring or activity scheduling) and the extent of adherence on a rating scale ranging from 0 (*made no effort to begin assignment*) to 3 (*fully completed assignment*).
Hawley et al,[29] 2014	MBCT for depression ($N = 18$)	Mindfulness HPQ,[29] which indicated the frequency and duration of their formal, informal, and total mindfulness practice during treatment.
Kok et al,[72] 2014	CBT delivered by Internet ($N = 129$)	Authors defined adherence as the proportion of patients that started the first module who completed the final module
Sachsenweger et al,[23] 2015	CBT for depression ($N = 28$)	Homework Rating Scale-II[30]
Shawyer et al,[73] 2012	MCBT for bipolar I or II ($N = 204$)	MBCT-Adherence Scale[74]
Shirk et al,[75] 2013	CBT for depression ($N = 83$)	Homework adherence was coded from audio recordings of sessions 2 through 4, in random order, on a 7-point scale ranging from 0 (*no effort*) to 6 (*did more than expected, exceptional effort*). During these sessions, homework included mood and thought monitoring as well as monitoring and countering negative thoughts. Scores were summed across sessions 2 through 4 to provide an index of early homework adherence.
Songprakun & McCann,[76] 2012	Self-help/bibliotherapy for depression ($N = 56$)	Proportion of the treatment manual's reading and writing components completed (eg, half, three-quarters)

Abbreviations: BA, behavioral activation; CT, cognitive therapy; HPQ, Homework Practice Questionnaire.

incorporating homework assignments into their treatment protocols. In-depth manual analysis of the sample that reported details of homework adherence assessment in anxiety and depression treatment (78% and 32%, respectively) demonstrated that the use of measures to assess quantity of homework adherence was more common, and that measures to assess quality of homework adherence, or extent of engagement, or theoretically meaningful determinants of adherence were almost absent.[23,31,32] Clinician ratings of homework adherence were most often used, but almost always were based on patient self-report, rather than completed logs, worksheets, or diaries. Despite the growing number of studies adopting technology for the delivery of CBT and other treatments, global assessments of adherence were used, such as the number of completed modules, mostly without other quantitative information.

There is long-standing discussion on the problems of ensuring adherence in mental health treatments.[33,34] Many investigators have recognized the limitations and problems of relying on the quantity of homework completion alone.[9,27] Quantity of homework completion does not convey the learning or degree of skill acquisition from the adherence. Moreover, there is not a 1:1 ratio between quantity and quality, and there is emerging evidence that quality may have stronger relations with symptom change in some CBT contexts.[9,11]

Nevertheless, the use of measures to assess the quantity of homework adherence is not necessarily a problem. The wide use of quantity assessment in the literature may signify that more articles are using some form of statistical analysis to examine adherence-outcome relations, or to statistically control for rates of adherence in examination of main treatment effects. Problems arise regarding the implications of what the quantity of homework adherence means, and particularly in the context of depression treatment, whereby motivational factors are pronounced, there is a need to study engagement. Other useful assessments that may be more directly interpretable, as an adjunct to the quantity of homework adherence, include treatment appraisals and other beliefs about the homework, given the literature supporting health belief models in adherence.[35,36]

This study has some limitations. First, the authors' aim was to provide an update of recent literature published from 2011 to 2016 and excluded earlier studies. Second, no automated study identification can verify the accuracy of the studies identified. However, their in-depth manual assessment also ensured that studies included in the review were appropriate.

Overall, the authors do not suggest that the quantity of homework adherence assessment be abandoned. The precision and transparency in homework adherence assessment would benefit from increased reporting, in terms of further quantitative data to support clinician judgments such as completed logs and worksheets. Alternative assessments such as engagement and theoretically meaningful determinants of adherence may be warranted and relevant to the evaluation of change mechanisms in CBT and other therapies. Quantity of homework adherence alone is difficult to interpret and may be misleading because adherence, skill acquisition, and engagement are different concepts and clinician assessment of completed tasks may inaccurately represent effort without patient data. By default, unless an argument can be made that the quality or skills acquired from the homework are not important (eg, in some studies where sessions are devoted to skill acquisition and between-session homework is focused on practice or generalization), then the global and exclusive assessment of homework quantity should thus be avoided.

DISCLOSURES

Dr N. Kazantzis receives royalties from Guilford Publications, Inc, Springer Publishing, and Routledge Press (which includes royalties from books on the content of this research). Grant monies for various projects come from the US National Institute of Mental Health, US National Institutes of Health, Helen Macpherson Smith Trust, and Lottery Health Research. Consulting and honoraria during the past several years have come from the Aiglé Foundation (Argentina), Australian Psychological Society, Australian Association of Cognitive Behavior Therapies, Cektos (Denmark), Boston University, da Associação Juizforana de Estudantes de Psicologia (Brazil), Greek Association for Behavioral and Cognitive Psychotherapies, The Institute of Behavior Research and Therapies (Greece), the International Congress of Cognitive Psychotherapy, the New Zealand Psychological Society, the Turkish Association of Cognitive and Behavior Psychotherapy, the World Congress of Behavior and Cognitive Therapies, the University of Crete, and various Australian universities. The other authors do not have any disclosures.

REFERENCES

1. Cuijpers P. Four decades of outcome research on psychotherapies for adult depression: an overview of a series of meta-analyses. Can Psychol 2017;58(1): 7–19.
2. Hofmann SG, Asnaani A, Vonk IJJ, et al. The efficacy of cognitive behaviour therapy: a review of meta-analyses. Cognit Ther Res 2012;36(5):427–40.
3. Tolin DF. Is CBT more effective than other therapies? A meta-analytic review. Clin Psychol Rev 2010;30(6):710–20.
4. Cuijpers P, Berking M, Andersson G, et al. A meta-analysis of cognitive-behavioural therapy for adult depression, alone and in comparison with other treatments. Can J Psychiatry 2013;58(7):376–85.
5. van Ballegooijen W, Cuijpers P, van Straten A, et al. Adherence to internet-based and face-to-face cognitive behavioural therapy for depression: a meta-analysis. PLoS One 2014;9(1):e100674.
6. Fernandez E, Salem D, Swift JK, et al. Meta-analysis of dropout from cognitive behavioral therapy: magnitude, timing, and moderators. J Consult Clin Psychol 2015;83(6):1108–22.
7. Hoelscher TJ, Lichstein KL, Rosenthal TL. Objective versus subjective assessment of relaxation compliance in anxious individuals. Behav Res Ther 1984;22: 187–93.
8. Kornblith SJ, Rehm LP, O'Hara MW, et al. The contribution of self-reinforcement training and behavioral assignments to the efficacy of self-control therapy for depression. Cognit Ther Res 1983;7:499–528.
9. Neimeyer RA, Kazantzis N, Kassler DM, et al. Group cognitive behavioural therapy for depression outcomes predicted by willingness to engage in homework, compliance with homework, and cognitive restructuring skill acquisition. Cogn Behav Ther 2008;37:199–215.
10. Kazantzis N, Deane FP, Ronan KR. Assessing compliance with homework assignments. J Clin Psychol 2004;60(6):627–41.
11. Kazantzis N, Whittington C, Zelencich L, et al. Quantity and quality of homework compliance: a meta-analysis of relations with outcome in cognitive behaviour therapy. Behav Ther 2016;47:755–72.
12. Helbig-Lang S, Fehm L. Problems with homework in CBT: rare exception or rather frequent? Beh Cog Psychother 2004;32(3):291–301.
13. Di Bona L, Saxon D, Barkham M, et al. Predictors of patient non-attendance at improving access to psychological therapy services sites. J Affect Disord 2014;169:157–64.
14. Nelson DL, Castonguay LG, Barwick F. Directions for the integration of homework in practice. In: Kazantzis N, L'Abate L, editors. Handbook of homework assignments in psychotherapy. New York: Springer US; 2007. p. 425–44.
15. Kazantzis N, Petrik AM, Cummins A. Homework Assignments: Available at: http://www.commonlanguagepsychotherapy.org/index.php?id=76. Accessed December 6, 2016.
16. Kazantzis N, Deane FP, Ronan KR. Homework assignments in cognitive and behavioral therapy: a meta-analysis. Clin Psychol-Sci Pr 2000;7:189–202.

17. Mausbach BT, Moore R, Roesch S, et al. The relationship between homework compliance and therapy outcomes: An updated meta-analysis. Cognit Ther Res 2010;34:429–38.
18. Kazantzis N, Whittington CJ, Dattilio FM. Meta-analysis of homework effects in cognitive and behavioural therapy: a replication and extension. Clin Psychol-Sci Pr 2010;17:144–56.
19. Burns DD, Spangler DL. Does psychotherapy homework lead to improvements in depression in CBT or does improvement lead to increased homework compliance? J Consult Clin Psychol 2000;69(6):1079–83.
20. Kazantzis N, Ronan KR, Deane FP. Concluding causation from correlation: comment on Burns and Spangler (2000). J Consult Clin Psychol 2001;69(6): 1079–83.
21. Wucherpfennig F, Rubel JA, Hollon SD, et al. Sudden gains in routine care cognitive behavioral therapy for depression: a replication with extensions. Behav Res Ther 2017;89:24–32.
22. Kazantzis N, Dattilio FM. Definitions of homework, types of homework, and ratings of the importance of homework among psychologists with cognitive behavior therapy and psychoanalytical theoretical orientations. J Clin Psychol 2010; 66(7):758–73.
23. Sachsenweger MA, Fletcher RB, Clarke D. Pessimism and homework in CBT for depression. J Clin Psychol 2015;71:1153–72.
24. Dozois DJA. Understanding and enhancing the effects of homework in cognitive-behavioral therapy. Clin Psychol-Sci Pr 2010;17(2):157–61.
25. Schmidt NB, Woolaway-Bickel K. The effects of treatment compliance on outcome in cognitive-behavioral therapy for panic disorder: quality versus quantity. J Consult Clin Psychol 2000;68(1):13–8.
26. Simpson HB, Maher M, Page JR, et al. Development of a patient adherence scale for exposure and response prevention therapy. Behav Ther 2010;41(1):30–7.
27. Primakoff L, Epstein N, Covi L. Homework compliance: an uncontrolled variable in cognitive therapy outcome research. Behav Ther 1986;17:433–46.
28. Campbell-Sills L, Barlow DH, Brown TA, et al. Effects of suppression and acceptance on emotional responses on individuals with anxiety and mood disorders. Behav Res Ther 2006;44:1251–63.
29. Hawley LL, Schwartz D, Bieling PJ, et al. Mindfulness practice, rumination and clinical outcome in mindfulness-based treatment. Cognit Ther Res 2014;38(1):1.
30. Kazantzis N, Deane FP, Ronan KR, et al, editors. Using homework assignments in cognitive behavior therapy. New York: Routledge; 2005. p. 61–72.
31. Hajda M, Kamaradova D, Latalova K, et al. Self-stigma, treatment adherence, a medication discontinuation in patients with bipolar disorders in remission – a cross sectional study. Act Nerv Sup Rediva 2015;57(1–2):6–11.
32. Klein NS, van Rijsbergen GD, Ten Doesschate MC, et al. Beliefs about the causes of depression and recovery and their impact on adherence, dosage, and successful tapering of antidepressants. Depress Anxiety 2017;34(3):227–35.
33. Nieuwlaat R, Wilczynski N, Navarro T, et al. Interventions for enhancing medication adherence. Cochrane Database Syst Rev 2014;(11):CD000011.
34. Haynes RB, Ackloo E, Sahota N, et al. Interventions for enhancing medication adherence. Cochrane Database Syst Rev 2008;(2):CD000011.
35. Scott J. Using health belief models to understand the efficacy-effectiveness gap for mood stabilizer treatments. Neuropsychobiology 2002;46:13–5.
36. Strauman TJ. Self-regulation and psychopathology: towards an integrative translational research paradigm. Annu Rev Clin Pschol 2017;13:497–523.

37. Alex Brake C, Sauer-Zavala S, Boswell JF, et al. Mindfulness-based exposure strategies as a transdiagnostic mechanism of change: an exploratory alternating treatment design. Behav Ther 2016;47(2):225–38.
38. Anand N, Sudhir PM, Math SB, et al. Cognitive behavior therapy in medication non-responders with obsessive–compulsive disorder: a prospective 1-year follow-up study. J Anxiety Disord 2011;25(7):939–45.
39. Andersson E, Ljótsson B, Hedman E, et al. Internet-based cognitive behavior therapy for obsessive compulsive disorder: a pilot study. BMC Psychiatry 2011; 11:125.
40. Aviram A, Westra HA. The impact of motivational interviewing on resistance in cognitive behavioural therapy for generalized anxiety disorder. Psychother Res 2011;21(6):698–708.
41. Bluett EJ, Zoellner LA, Feeny NC. Does change in distress matter? Mechanisms of change in prolonged exposure for PTSD. J Behav Ther Exp Psychiatry 2014; 45(1):97–104.
42. Brown AJ, Bollini AM, Craighead LW, et al. Self-monitoring of reexperiencing symptoms: a randomized trial. J Trauma Stress 2014;27(5):519–25.
43. Cammin-Nowak S, Helbig-Lang S, Lang T, et al. Specificity of homework compliance effects on treatment outcome in CBT: evidence from a controlled trial on panic disorder and agoraphobia. J Clin Psychol 2013;69(6):616–29.
44. Chavira DA, Golinelli D, Sherbourne C, et al. Treatment engagement and response to CBT among Latinos with anxiety disorders in primary care. J Consult Clin Psychol 2014;82(3):392–403.
45. Cooper AA, Kline AC, Graham B, et al. Homework "dose," type, and helpfulness as predictors of clinical outcomes in prolonged exposure for PTSD. Behav Ther 2016;48(2):182–94.
46. Dear BF, Titov N, Schwencke G, et al. An open trial of a brief transdiagnostic internet treatment for anxiety and depression, vol. 49. Netherlands: Elsevier Science; 2011. p. 830–7.
47. De Kleine RA, Hendriks GJ, Kusters WJC, et al. A randomized placebo-controlled trial of D-cycloserine to enhance exposure therapy for posttraumatic stress disorder. Biol Psychiatry 2012;71(11):962–8.
48. Dowling N, Thomas N, Blair-West S, et al. Intensive residential treatment for obsessive-compulsive disorder: outcomes and predictors of patient adherence to cognitive-behavioural therapy. J Obsessive Compuls Relat Disord 2016;9: 82–9.
49. Gershkovich M, Herbert JD, Forman EM, et al. Guided internet-based self-help intervention for social anxiety disorder with videoconferenced therapist support. Cogn Behav Pract 2016;23(2):239–55.
50. Glenn D, Golinelli D, Rose RD, et al. Who gets the most out of cognitive behavioral therapy for anxiety disorders? The role of treatment dose and patient engagement. J Consult Clin Psychol 2013;81(4):639–49.
51. Gloster AT, Wittchen H-U, Einsle F, et al. Psychological treatment for panic disorder with agoraphobia: a randomized controlled trial to examine the role of therapist-guided exposure in situ in CBT. J Consult Clin Psychol 2011;79(3): 406–20.
52. Hundt NE, Amspoker AB, Kraus-Schuman C, et al. Predictors of CBT outcome in older adults with GAD. J Anxiety Disord 2014;28(8):845–50.
53. King AP, Erickson TM, Giardino ND, et al. A pilot study of group mindfulness-based cognitive therapy (MBCT) for combat veterans with posttraumatic stress disorder (PTSD). Depress Anxiety 2013;30(7):638–45.

54. Lebeau RT, Davies CD, Culver NC, et al. Homework compliance counts in cognitive-behavioral therapy. Cogn Behav Ther 2013;42(3):171–9.
55. Lewin AB, Peris TS, Bergman R, et al. The role of treatment expectancy in youth receiving exposure-based CBT for obsessive compulsive disorder. Behav Res Ther 2011;49(9):536–43.
56. Mataix-Cols D, Turner C, Monzani B, et al. Cognitive-behavioural therapy with post-session D-cycloserine augmentation for paediatric obsessive-compulsive disorder: pilot randomised controlled trial. Br J Psychiatry 2014;204(1):77–8.
57. Meuret AE, Twohig MP, Rosenfield D, et al. Brief acceptance and commitment therapy and exposure for panic disorder: a pilot study. Cogn Behav Pract 2012;19(4):606–18.
58. Milrod B, Chambless DL, Gallop R, et al. Psychotherapies for panic disorder: a tale of two sites. J Clin Psychiatry 2016;77(7):927–35.
59. Olatunji BO, Rosenfield D, Monzani B, et al. Effects of homework compliance on cognitive-behavioral therapy with D-cycloserine augmentation for children with obsessive compulsive disorder. Depress Anxiety 2015;32(12):935–43.
60. Park JM, Small BJ, Geller DA, et al. Does D-cycloserine augmentation of CBT improve therapeutic homework compliance for pediatric obsessive-compulsive disorder? J Child Fam Stud 2014;23(5):863–71.
61. Ready DJ, Sylvers P, Worley V, et al. The impact of group-based exposure therapy on the PTSD and depression of 30 combat veterans. Psychol Trauma 2012; 4(1):84–93.
62. Robinson S, Turner C, Heyman I, et al. The feasibility and acceptability of a cognitive-behavioural self-help intervention for adolescents with obsessive-compulsive disorder. Cogn Behav Ther 2013;41(1):117–22.
63. Simpson HB, Maher MJ, Wang Y, et al. Patient adherence predicts outcome from cognitive behavioral therapy in obsessive-compulsive disorder. J Consult Clin Psychol 2011;79(2):247–52.
64. Westra HA. Comparing the predictive capacity of observed in-session resistance to self-reported motivation in cognitive behavioral therapy. Behav Res Ther 2011; 49(2):106–13.
65. Wetherell JL, Johnson K, Chang D, et al. Activity, balance, learning, and exposure (ABLE): a new intervention for fear of falling. Int J Geriatr Psychiatry 2016;31(7): 791–8.
66. Wheaton MG, Galfalvy H, Steinman SA, et al. Patient adherence and treatment outcome with exposure and response prevention for OCD: which components of adherence matter and who becomes well? Behav Res Ther 2016;85:6–12.
67. Zargar F, Farid AAA, Atef-Vahid MK, et al. Comparing the effectiveness of acceptance-based behavior therapy and applied relaxation on acceptance of internal experiences, engagement in valued actions and quality of life in generalized anxiety disorder. J Res Med Sci 2013;18(2):118–22.
68. Wilson KG, Sandoz EK, Kitchens J, et al. The valued living questionnaire: defining and measuring valued action within a behavioral framework. Psychol Rec 2010; 60:249–72.
69. Zou JB, Dear BF, Titov N, et al. Brief internet-delivered cognitive behavioral therapy for anxiety in older adults: a feasibility trial. J Anxiety Disord 2012;26(6): 650–5.
70. Conklin LR, Strunk DR. A session-to-session examination of homework engagement in cognitive therapy for depression: do patients experience immediate benefits?, vol. 72. Netherlands: Elsevier Science; 2015. p. 56–62.

71. Folke F, Hursti T, Tungström S, et al. Behavioral activation between acute inpatient and outpatient psychiatry: description of a protocol and a pilot feasibility study, vol. 22. Netherlands: Elsevier Science; 2015. p. 468–80.
72. Kok G, Bockting C, Burger H, et al. Mobile cognitive therapy: adherence and acceptability of an online intervention in remitted recurrently depressed patients. Internet Interv 2014;1(2):65–73.
73. Shawyer F, Meadows GN, Judd F, et al. The DARE study of relapse prevention in depression: design for a phase 1/2 translational randomised controlled trial involving mindfulness-based cognitive therapy and supported self monitoring. BMC Psychiatry 2012;12:3.
74. Segal ZV, Teasdale JD, Williams JMG, et al. The Mindfulness-Based Cognitive Therapy Adherence Scale: inter-rater reliability, adherence to protocol and treatment distinctiveness. Clin Psychol Psychother 2002;9:131–8.
75. Shirk SR, Crisostomo PS, Jungbluth N, et al. Cognitive mechanisms of change in CBT for adolescent depression: associations among client involvement, cognitive distortions, and treatment outcome. Int J Cogn Ther 2013;6(4):311–24.
76. Songprakun W, McCann TV. Effectiveness of a self-help manual on the promotion of resilience in individuals with depression in Thailand: a randomised controlled trial, vol. 12. United Kingdom: BioMed Central Limited; 2012.

The Effect of Cognitive Behavioral Interventions on Depression and Anxiety Symptoms in Patients with Schizophrenia Spectrum Disorders: A Systematic Review

Sandra M. Opoka, MSc*, Tania M. Lincoln, PhD

KEYWORDS

• Psychosis • Schizophrenia • Anxiety • Depression • CBT • PTSD

KEY POINTS

- Depression and anxiety are comorbid disorders in patients with psychosis; symptoms of depression and anxiety are relevant for the formation and maintenance of psychotic symptoms.
- A systematic review of cognitive–behavioral interventions aimed at anxiety and depression in people with psychosis identified 14 studies investigating a heterogeneous set of interventions.
- The studies indicated a positive intervention effect on symptom severity with medium-to-large controlled effects for depression, small-to-large controlled effects for anxiety, and medium-to-large controlled effects for posttraumatic stress disorder.
- Only a few studies reported a reduction of psychotic symptoms and the effect sizes among these studies ranged considerably.
- Comorbid depression and anxiety can be treated successfully, but further research is needed to examine whether and under which conditions the effects carry over to psychotic symptoms.

INTRODUCTION

High comorbidity rates are found among patients with schizophrenia spectrum disorders, with prevalence rates of up to 50% for depression, 38% for anxiety disorders, and 29% for PTSD. Such comorbidities are associated with more severe symptom

Disclosures: None.
Clinical Psychology and Psychotherapy, Institut of Psychology, Universität Hamburg, Von-Melle-Park-5, Hamburg 20146, Germany
* Corresponding author.
E-mail address: sandra.martha.opoka@uni-hamburg.de

Psychiatr Clin N Am 40 (2017) 641–659
http://dx.doi.org/10.1016/j.psc.2017.08.005
0193-953X/17/© 2017 Elsevier Inc. All rights reserved.

psych.theclinics.com

Abbreviations	
ADAPT	Acceptance-based depression and psychosis therapy
CBTp	Cognitive–behavioral therapy for psychosis
COMET	Competitive memory training
EMDR	Eye movement desensitization and reprocessing
PE	Prolonged exposure
PMR	Progressive muscle relaxation
PTSD	Posttraumatic stress disorder
TAU	Treatment-as-usual

expression and poorer prognosis.[1,2] Even where the diagnostic criteria for comorbid depression, anxiety, or PTSD are not met, patients tend to display at least some related symptoms or issues such as low self-esteem, worrying and rumination, lack of self-efficacy, hyperarousal, sleep disturbances, or lack of motivation.[3–8]

Not only do negative affective states add to the already high level of distress in patients with psychosis, they are also relevant to the formation and maintenance of psychotic symptoms.[9,10] Garety and colleagues[11] introduced a cognitive model to explain the formation of positive symptoms of psychosis, postulating that positive symptoms, such as delusions, arise from the way vulnerable individuals interpret stressful experiences and that this interpretation is influenced by the affective state. Numerous studies support both the postulated link between negative affect and psychotic symptoms and the mediating function of negative affect between stressors and psychotic symptoms. For example, symptoms of depression have been found to be associated with and predict increased auditory hallucinations and persecutory delusions,[5,12,13] and to serve as a mediator between external stressors and paranoia.[14,15] Similarly, worry has been shown to predict the occurrence and persistence of subclinical paranoia and delusions,[16–18] the induction of state anxiety to increase paranoid ideation[19,20] and anxiety to mediate the effect of stressors on paranoia.[15] Moreover, studies have found depression to impact on how patients with psychosis cope with psychotic symptoms. For example, Lincoln and colleagues[21] found that, in comparison with healthy individuals, patients with psychosis respond to paranoid beliefs in a more dysfunctional manner,[22] such as feeling tensed, guilty, and responsible, which is largely explained by their higher levels of depression. Hence, empirical evidence suggests that addressing depression and anxiety as a therapeutic target is relevant to psychosis and is likely to have a positive impact on positive symptoms.

Over the last decades specific cognitive–behavioral interventions have been developed for psychosis.[23] Cognitive–behavioral therapy for psychosis (CBTp) shares many elements of cognitive–behavioral interventions for other disorders, such as working with case formulations, improving behavioral skills, and challenging dysfunctional beliefs about the self. The elements that are specific to psychosis involve developing and improving coping strategies for psychotic symptoms, and cognitive restructuring of delusional beliefs and dysfunctional beliefs about symptoms.[24] In recent years, CBTp has been extensively evaluated and is now recommended in many national guidelines for psychosis (eg, German Association for Psychiatry, Psychotherapy and Neurology[25] and National Institute for Health and Care Excellence[26]). However, CBTp is a complex and individualized approach, requiring intensive training, to which not all therapists seem to have access.[27–29] This limits its application in practice. In contrast, all CBT-trained therapists are familiar with interventions targeting depression and anxiety. If such regular interventions can be shown to affect psychotic symptoms by reducing depression and anxiety in patients with psychosis, this could add to solving the implementation problem of CBTp.

Another aspect is that not all patients willingly accept the label of schizophrenia. This is often termed "low insight" and has been associated with low treatment adherence.[4] In contrast, affective problems present a more relevant treatment goal for many patients,[30] who might thus be more willing to accept interventions targeting anxiety or depression.

Tying it all together, symptoms of depression and anxiety are common in patients with psychosis and previous research has ascertained negative affect to be critical to the formation and maintenance of psychotic symptoms. Although CBTp has been found to be effective, its implementation has been challenging so far. In contrast, interventions focusing on depression and anxiety are familiar to most therapists, are more broadly implemented, and are likely to be more acceptable to some patients. Examining the effectiveness of CBT-based interventions that focus specifically on symptoms of depression and anxiety symptoms as well as the impact these interventions have on psychotic symptoms might thus add to solving the implementation problem at hand. Herein, we provide a systematic overview on the existing studies in this field to synthesize what is known and derive directions for further research in this field.

METHODS

Suitable peer-reviewed articles in English were identified in January 2017 by conducting 2 separate literature searches (depression and anxiety focused[a]) in electronic databases (MEDLINE and PsycINFO) via Ovid. The following search terms were used: ("CBT", "cognitive behavio*", "cognitive-behavio*", "intervention", "therapy", or "training" or "treat*" or "effect*" or "randomized clinical trial") were combined with ("schizophren*", "psychosis", "psychotic", "delusion*", or "hallucination*"). In addition, the search terms ("depress*" or "mood") were included within the depression-focused search and ("anxiety", "phobi*", "PTSD", "posttraumatic stress disorder", "post traumatic stress disorder", "posttraumatic stress disorder", "panic" or "worry") within the anxiety-focused search. In the second and third steps, titles followed by abstracts were screened for relevance. The remaining articles were examined in detail regarding predefined inclusion and exclusion criteria. Inclusion criteria encompassed (a) English studies describing (b) randomized controlled trials examining the effect of (c) CBT-based interventions focusing on (d) depressive, anxiety, or PTSD symptoms as the main outcome in (e) patients diagnosed with schizophrenia spectrum disorders. Exclusion criteria were (a) subclinical or at-risk samples regarding psychotic diagnosis and (b) studies using diagnostic systems older than *Diagnostic and Statistical Manual of Mental Disorders*, fourth edition, or the *International Classification of Diseases,* 10th edition. Controlled effect sizes reported in this review are based on those reported in the original studies and include effect sizes based on the postassessment differences between the intervention and the control group with or without controlling for preassessment scores. Where controlled effect sizes were not reported but mean values and standard deviations were provided,[31-33] the effect sizes were calculated by subtracting the posttreatment mean of the control group from the mean of the intervention group and dividing it by the pooled standard deviation. Moreover, the authors of studies not reporting results on psychotic symptoms[31,32,34-37] were contacted for additional information, which was provided in 2 cases.[32,34]

---

[a] Until recently, PTSD was grouped together with anxiety disorders in *Diagnostic and Statistical Manual of Mental Disorders,* 4th edition. Although, we acknowledge that they comprise a distinct category in the *Diagnostic and Statistical Manual of Mental Disorders,* 5the edition, we have subsumed them within the anxiety category for pragmatic reasons in this review.

RESULTS

The literature search revealed a total of 483 peer-reviewed studies that specifically examined the effect of CBT-based interventions on depression and 105 studies that focused on anxiety related problems, including PTSD. Of those, 6 studies on depression and 8 studies on anxiety met the inclusion criteria. A detailed overview of the study selection process is presented in **Fig. 1**.

Of the 6 studies focusing on depression, one used a waitlist control group, 2 used treatment-as-usual (TAU) control groups, 1 used a placebo control group (eg, enhanced assessment and monitoring), and 2 studies used active control groups (eg, social skills and occupational therapy). Of those studies focusing on anxiety, 3 used waitlist control groups, 2 used TAU, and 3 used a placebo control condition (eg, reading in therapy room). Intervention effects on psychotic symptoms were reported in 5 of 6 studies focusing on depression and in 4 of 8 studies focusing on anxiety. The mean dropout rate was 14.8% (range, 0%–30.8%). Details on sample sizes, target population, therapy format, measurement time points, outcome measures, effects sizes, and dropout rates are provided in **Tables 1** and **2**. We provide a brief summary of the design, the interventions, and the main results of each of the selected studies.

Depression

Cognitive–behavioral interventions focusing on self-esteem

In a pilot trial, Freeman and colleagues[38] investigated the effect of a brief cognitive–behavioral intervention focused on normalizing and reviewing negative thoughts about the self and enhancing positive activities. A small controlled effect size was found for the reduction of negative beliefs about the self in comparison with TAU, but the differences between groups were nonsignificant. Overall, symptoms of depression decreased significantly with a medium-to-large controlled effect size for the difference between the treatment and the control group at the post-treatment assessment, but the benefits were not maintained at follow-up. Medium-to-large but nonsignificant controlled effect sizes were reported for paranoia and delusions.

Memory trainings

Van der Gaag and colleagues[39] examined competitive memory training (COMET), in which memories associated with positive self-esteem were retrieved and strengthened. The activation of this positive self-image was used to weaken the negative content of voices and enhance self-confidence. The results indicated a positive effect of COMET on depressive symptoms compared with TAU. The controlled effect size was medium to large. This intervention effect was fully mediated by self-esteem and acceptance of voices and partially mediated by the attributed power to the voices and the social ranking of oneself in relation to the voices. COMET did not affect the total score for auditory hallucinations, but a medium controlled effect size was reported for the cognitive interpretation of voices.

Ricarte and colleagues[36] investigated a group-based, event-specific memory training compared with an active control group (social skills and occupational therapy). The patients were instructed to write diary entries focusing on specific daily events and their emotional implications, as well as autobiographical memories. The study found a significant improvement in depressive symptoms within the intervention group, whereas there were no changes within the active control group. The controlled effect size was large. No results were reported for psychotic symptoms.

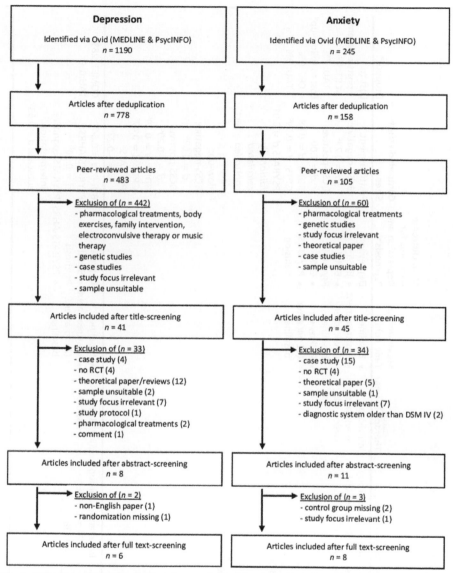

Fig. 1. Selection of studies. DSM, *Diagnostic and Statistical Manual of Mental Disorders*; RCT, randomized-controlled trial.

Mindfulness and acceptance-based interventions

In a pilot trial, Gaudiano and colleagues[40] compared an acceptance-based depression and psychosis therapy (ADAPT) with a placebo control group (enhanced assessment and monitoring). ADAPT included rapport building, identification of values and goals, and behavior activation, as well as mindfulness and acceptance skills. The controlled effect size for depressive symptoms was large. However, the controlled effect for the group difference in psychotic symptoms was small.

Moritz and colleagues[41] compared an online mindfulness intervention to an active control group (online progressive muscle relaxation [PMR]). In both interventions,

Table 1
Details on reviewed studies with focus on depression

Reference	n	Patient Population	Intervention (n)	Therapy Format	Measurement Time Points	Main Outcome Measures for Depression and Psychosis	Controlled Effect Sizes	Dropout[a]
Freeman et al,[38] 2014	30	Patients (18–70 y) with a diagnosis of schizophrenia, schizoaffective disorder, or delusional disorder and negative beliefs about the self and current persecutory delusions; stable on medication	Intervention group (15) = brief CBT; TAU (15)	Individual; 6 sessions over 8 wk	• Baseline • Posttreatment (8 wk after baseline) • Follow-up (12 wk after baseline)	Depression • BCSS • BDI-II Psychosis • GPTS • PSYRATS-delusion	Posttreatment: BCSS-negative: $d = 0.24^c$ BCSS-positive: $d = 1.00$ BDI-II: $d = 0.68$ GPTS: $d = 0.59^c$ PSYRATS $d = 0.91^c$ *Additionally calculated controlled effect sizes* Follow-up: BCSS-negative: $d = 0.09^c$ BCSS-positive: $d = -0.20^c$ BDI-II: $d = 0.39^c$ GPTS: $d = 0.47^c$ PSYRATS $d = -0.27^c$	Lost to posttreatment[e] CBT: 0% TAU: 7% Lost to follow-up[e] CBT: 0% TAU: 0%
van der Gaag et al,[39] 2012	77	Patients with schizophrenia-spectrum disorder and persistent auditory hallucinations	Intervention group (39) = COMET; TAU (38)	Individual; 7 sessions	• Baseline • Posttreatment (2 mo after baseline)	Depression • BDI-II Psychosis • PSYRATS-AHRS	BDI-II: $d = 0.64^b$ PSYRATS-AHRS: $d = 0.30^{b,c}$ PSYRATS-cognitive interpretation subscale: $d = 0.63^b$	COMET: 28% TAU: 0%

Study	N	Sample	Groups	Format	Assessment	Outcomes	Results	Dropout
Ricarte et al,[36] 2012	53	Inpatients and outpatients with a diagnosis of schizophrenia; clinically stable	Intervention group (24) = event-specific memory training; Active control group (26) = social skills and occupational therapy	Group (8–10 participants); 10 weekly sessions; 90 min/session	• Baseline • Posttreatment (1 wk after final session)	Depression • BDI Psychosis • BPRS • PANSS	BDI: $\eta^2_{partial} = 0.21$ No results on psychotic symptoms reported	Intervention: 8% Control: 4%
Gaudiano,[40] 2015	13	Outpatients (≥18 y; recruited while inpatients) on medication with a diagnosis of a severe major depressive disorder with psychotic features or schizoaffective disorder/depressive type	Intervention group (6) = ADAPT; Placebo control group (7) = enhanced assessment and monitoring	Individual; 16 sessions over 4 mo	• Baseline • Posttreatment (4 mo after baseline) • Follow-up (7 mo after baseline)	Depression • QIDS-C Psychosis • BPRS	Posttreatment: QIDS-C: $d = 0.81$ [b,d] (ITT: $d = 0.86$) [b,d] BPRS: $d = 0.06$ [b,d] (ITT: $d = 0.29$) [b,d] *Additionally calculated controlled effect sizes* Follow-up: QIDS-C: $d = 4.58$ [b,d] (ITT: $d = 0.85$) [b,d] BPRS: $d = 0.12$ [b,d] (ITT: $d = -0.47$) [b,d]	Lost to posttreatment: ADAPT: 17% EAM: 43% Lost to follow-up: ADAPT: 40% EAM: 0%
Moritz et al,[41] 2015	90	Outpatients (18–65 y) with a diagnosis of schizophrenia	Intervention group (38) = self-help mindfulness; Active control group (52) = PMR	Individual; self-help manual and audio files over 6 wk	• Baseline • Posttreatment (6 wk after baseline)	Depression • CES-D Psychosis • Paranoia Checklist	CES-D: $\eta^2_{partial} < 0.001$ [c] Paranoia Checklist: $\eta^2_{partial} = 0.002$ [c]	Mindfulness: 26% PMR: 31%

(continued on next page)

Table 1
(continued)

Reference	n	Patient Population	Intervention (n)	Therapy Format	Measurement Time Points	Main Outcome Measures for Depression and Psychosis	Controlled Effect Sizes	Dropout[a]
Moritz et al,[42] 2016	58	Outpatients (18–65 y) with a diagnosis of schizophrenia and subjective depressive symptoms	Intervention group (31) = online depression intervention (HelpID) Waitlist control group (27)	Individual; 12 weekly modules; 45–60 min/module	• Baseline • Posttreatment (3 mo after baseline)	Depression • CES-D • PHQ-9 • PANSS (item 6) Psychosis • Paranoia Checklist • PANSS distress subscale	CES-D: $\eta^2_{partial}$ = 0.18 PHQ-9: $\eta^2_{partial}$ = 0.08[c] PANSS (item 6): $\eta^2_{partial}$ = 0.10 Paranoia Checklist: $\eta^2_{partial}$ < 0.001[c] PANSS distress subscale: $\eta^2_{partial}$ = 0.08[c]	Intervention: 19%[e] Waitlist: 11%[e]

Abbreviations: ADAPT, Acceptance-based Depression and Psychosis Therapy; BCSS, Brief Core Schema Scale; BDI, Beck Depression Inventory; BDI-II, Beck Depression Inventory II; BPRS, Brief Psychiatric Rating Scale; CBT, cognitive–behavioral therapy; CES-D, Center for Epidemiologic Studies - Depression Scale; COMET, competitive memory training; EAM, enhanced assessment and monitoring; GPTS, Green et al Paranoid Thoughts Scale; ITT, intention-to-treat; PANSS, Positive and Negative Syndrome Scale for Schizophrenia; PHQ-9, Patient-Health-Questionnaire-9; PMR, progressive muscle relaxation; PSYRATS-AHRS, Psychosis Rating Scales-Auditory Hallucination Rating Scale; QIDS-C, quick inventory of depressive symptomatology-clinician; TAU, treatment as usual/standard care.

[a] For better comparability, information on dropout given by authors were converted in percent.

[b] Precise formula for the computation of effect sizes is not provided.

[c] Nonsignificant effect size.

[d] No information on significance of effect.

[e] Additionally calculated from flowchart (lost from randomization to posttreatment; lost from randomization to follow-up).

the participants received a self-help manual including an introduction to the concept and a description of the exercises as well as accompanying audio files. In both groups, depression reduced significantly, but no intervention was superior to the other. No significant change was observed for psychotic symptoms, neither within nor between the groups.

Integrative intervention packages

Another study by Moritz and colleagues[42] examined an Internet intervention called Help-ID compared with a waitlist control group. The methods used within this program were based on CBT, acceptance and commitment therapy, and systemic therapy, and also included other techniques such as relaxation exercises and music therapy. A significant group difference was found for symptom decrease on 2 of 3 depression measures within the intervention group relative to the control group. The controlled effect sizes were in the medium-to-large range. The reported controlled effect sizes for psychotic symptoms were below the small range and nonsignificant.

Anxiety

Relaxation

Chen and colleagues[31] examined the effect of daily PMR sessions over an 11-day period. The results indicate a significant decrease in anxiety score with a large additionally calculated controlled effect size for the difference between the treatment and the control group (sitting quietly in therapy room) at the posttreatment assessment. However, the controlled group difference was only marginally significant at the 1-week follow-up. No information regarding posttreatment psychotic symptoms was reported.

Vancampfort and colleagues[34] examined the effect of a single PMR session on state anxiety, which reduced significantly in the intervention group, but not in the placebo control condition (sitting quietly or reading). The controlled effect size was large. Psychotic symptoms were only examined at pretreatment.

Georgiev and colleagues[35] replicated the study by Vancampfort and colleagues,[34] examining the effect of a single PMR session on state anxiety, which decreased significantly in the intervention group, but not in the placebo control condition (sitting quietly or reading). The controlled effect size was small. No data were collected on psychotic symptoms.

Cognitive–behavioral interventions for social anxiety

In a pilot trial, Halperin and colleagues[32] examined a group-based cognitive–behavioral intervention for social anxiety, including psychoeducation, exposure, cognitive restructuring, and role plays. They found a significant improvement of anxiety within the intervention group compared with no or little change in the waitlist control group. Additionally calculated controlled effect sizes were in the small range. Individual gains were maintained over a 6-week period. No specific measures of psychotic symptoms were administered. Because the authors administered the Brief Symptom Inventory, information on the psychotic symptom subscale was gained via personal communication (David Castle, 2017), indicating no reduction compared with waitlist controls.

Kingsep and colleagues[37] evaluated a cognitive–behavioral group program, encompassing psychoeducation, exposition, cognitive restructuring, and role plays. They found a positive intervention effect on social anxiety compared with a waitlist control group at the posttreatment assessment with a medium-to-large controlled effect size. Improvement was maintained at the 2-month follow-up. No specific measures of psychotic symptoms were administered.

Table 2
Details on reviewed studies with a focus on anxiety

Reference	N	Patient Population	Intervention (n)	Therapy Format	Measurement Time Points	Main Outcome Measures for Anxiety and Psychosis	Controlled Effect Sizes	Dropout[b]
Chen et al,[31] 2009	18	Inpatients with a diagnosis of schizophrenia and a significant level of anxiety willing to accept treatment with a limited number of atypical antipsychotics	Intervention group (9) = PMR Placebo control group (9) = sitting quietly in therapy room	Group (9 participants); 1 training session + 11 sessions on 11 consecutive days	• Baseline • Posttreatment (11 d after first intervention-session) • Follow-up (1 wk after finalization of intervention)	Anxiety • BAI Psychosis • SAPS	*Additionally calculated controlled effect sizes* Posttreatment: BAI: $d = 1.43$[a] SAPS: not enough data available for calculation[c] Follow-up: Not enough data available for calculation[c]	Lost to posttreatment PMR: 11% Control: 33%[d] Lost to follow-up No information
Vancampfort et al,[34] 2011	64	Inpatients with a diagnosis of schizophrenia	Intervention group (27) = PMR Placebo control group (26) = sitting quietly/reading	2 weekly sessions of habituation; testing session in the third week; 25 minutes/session	• Baseline: 5 minutes before intervention • Post-treatment (immediately after completion of condition)	Anxiety • STAI	STAI: $d = -1.25$	PMR: 16% Control: 19%
Georgiev et al,[35] 2012	64	Chronic patients with a diagnosis of schizophrenia; remitted acute symptoms	Intervention group (27) = PMR Placebo control group (26) = sitting quietly/reading	2 weekly sessions of habituation; testing session in third week; 25 minutes/session	• Baseline: 5 minutes before intervention • Posttreatment (immediately after completion of condition)	Anxiety • STAI	STAI: $d = -0.22$	PMR: 3% Control: 6%[e]

Study	N	Population	Intervention	Format	Assessment	Measures	Results	Dropout
Halperin et al,[32] 2000	20	Outpatients with a diagnosis of schizophrenia and a significant level of social anxiety	Intervention group (7) = group-based cognitive–behavioral intervention for social anxiety; Waitlist control group (9)	Group; 8 weekly sessions; 2 h/session	• Baseline • Posttreatment • Follow-up (6 wk posttreatment)	Anxiety • BSPS • SIAS; Psychosis • BSI	*Additionally calculated controlled effect sizes* Posttreatment: BSPS: d = −0.11; SIAS: d = 0.30; BSI: no data available on relevant subscale; Follow-up: Not enough data available	Intervention: 30% Control: 20%
Kingsep et al,[37] 2003	33	Patients with a diagnosis of schizophrenia and comorbid social anxiety	Intervention group (16) = cognitive–behavioral group treatment; Waitlist control group (17)	Group; 12 weekly sessions + 1 follow-up session (2 months after last treatment session); 2 h/session	• Baseline • Posttreatment • Follow-up (2 mo posttreatment)	Anxiety • BSPS • SIAS • BFNE; Psychosis • BSI	Posttreatment: Anxiety mean: d = 0.64; SIAS: d = 0.69; BSPS: d = 0.17; BFNE: d = 1.05; BSI: no data available on relevant subscale; Follow-up: Not enough data available	Total: 20%

(continued on next page)

Table 2
(continued)

Reference	N	Patient Population	Intervention (n)	Therapy Format	Measurement Time Points	Main Outcome Measures for Anxiety and Psychosis	Controlled Effect Sizes	Dropout[b]
Foster et al,[33] 2010	24	Inpatients and outpatients (18–65 y) with a diagnosis of schizophrenia, schizoaffective disorder, or delusional disorder having a significant level of worry and persistent persecutory delusions (>6 mo)	Intervention group (12) = W-CBT TAU (12)	Individual; 4 sessions over 1 month	• Baseline (before randomization) • End of treatment (1 mo after randomization) • Follow-up (2 mo after randomization)	Anxiety • PSWQ Psychosis • PSYRATS-delusions • GPTS	*Additionally calculated controlled effect sizes* Posttreatment: PSWQ: d = 0.57 PSYRATS-total: d = 0.94 GPTS-total: d = 0.09[d] Follow-up: PSWQ: d = 0.74 PSYRATS-total: d = 0.80 GPTS-total: d = 0.57[d]	Lost to posttreatment[d] W-CBT: 25% TAU: 8% Lost to follow-up[d] W-CBT: 17% TAU: 17%
Freeman et al,[43] 2015	150	Inpatients and outpatients (18–65 y) with a diagnosis of schizophrenia, schizoaffective disorder, or delusional disorder having a significant level of worry and current persecutory delusions; stable on medication	Intervention group (73) = CBT TAU (77)	Individual; 6 sessions over 8 wk; 1 h/session	• Baseline • Posttreatment (8 wk after baseline) • Follow-up (24 wk after baseline)	Anxiety • PSWQ Psychosis • PSYRATS • PANSS • GPTS	*Differences in average outcome across posttreatment and follow-up assessment* PSWQ: d = 0.47 PSYRATS: d = 0.49 PANSS: d = 0.42 GPTS: d = 0.45	Lost to posttreatment[d] CBT: 4% Control: 5% Lost to follow-up[d] CBT: 7% Control: 5%

| Van den Berg et al,[44] 2015 | 155 | Outpatients (18–65 years) with a diagnosis of a psychotic disorder or mood disorder with psychotic features and comorbid posttraumatic stress disorder | Intervention group (53) = PE Intervention group (55) = EMDR Waiting control group (47) | Individual; 8 sessions over 10 wk; 90 min/session | Baseline • Posttreatment (10 wk after baseline) • Follow-up (6 mo) | Anxiety • CAPS • PSS-SR Psychosis information retrieved from de Bont et al. (2016) • GPTS • PSYRATS-AHRS | PE vs WL (posttreatment) CAPS: d = 0.78 PSS-SR: d = 0.88 GPTS: d = 0.62 AHRS: d = 0.56[d] PE vs WL (follow-up) CAPS: d = 0.63 PSS-SR: d = 0.70 GPTS: d = 0.54 AHRS: d = −0.42[c] EMDR vs WL (posttreatment) CAPS: d = 0.65 PSS-SR: d = 0.85 GPTS: d = 0.59 AHRS: d = 0.40[d] EMDR vs WL (follow-up) CAPS: d = 0.53 PSS-SR: d = 0.70 GPTS: d = 0.33[c] AHRS: d = 0.06[c] | Discontinuation of treatment PE: 25% EMDR: 20% Lost to posttreatment[d] PE: 11% EMDR: 20% Control: 17% Lost to follow-up[d] PE: 15% EMDR: 22% Control: 15% |

Abbreviations: BAI, Beck Anxiety Inventory; BDI-II, Beck Depression Inventory II; BFNE, Brief Fear of Negative Evaluation Scale; BSI, Brief Symptom Inventory; BSPS, Brief Social Phobia Scale; CAPS, Clinician-Administered PTSD Scale; CBT, cognitive–behavioral therapy; CDSS, Calgary Depression Scale for Schizophrenia; EMDR, eye movement desensitization and reprocessing; GPTS, Green et al Paranoid Thoughts Scale; PANSS, Positive and Negative Syndrome Scale for Schizophrenia; PE, prolonged exposure; PMR, progressive muscle relaxation; PSS-SR, Posttraumatic Stress Symptom Scale Self-report; PSWQ, Penn State Worry Questionnaire; PSYRATS-AHRS, Psychosis Rating Scales-Auditory Hallucination Rating Scale; QIDS-C, Quick Inventory of Depressive Symptomatology-Clinician; SAPS, Scale for Assessment of Positive Symptoms; SIAS, Social Interaction Anxiety Scale; STAI, State Anxiety Inventory; TAU, treatment as usual/standard care; W-CBT, cognitive–behavioral worry intervention; WL, wait list.

[a] Effect size was additionally calculated based on the pooled standard deviation at baseline (follow-up standard deviation not available).
[b] For better comparability, information on dropout given by authors were converted in percent.
[c] Nonsignificant effect size.
[d] Additionally calculated from flow-chart (lost from randomization to posttreatment; lost from randomization to follow-up).
[e] Discrepant information: dropout within control group was 13% according to flow chart.

Cognitive–behavioral interventions for worry

A pilot trial by Foster and colleagues[33] investigated a worry-focused intervention that included psychoeducation, identification of individual triggers, implementation of worry periods, and relaxation exercises. Anxiety scores reduced within the intervention group at posttreatment compared with TAU and improvement was maintained at 2-month follow-up. The additionally calculated controlled effect sizes were medium at posttreatment and medium to large at follow-up. The results indicate a reduction in persecutory delusions, including the delusion distress, as measured with the delusion subscale of the Psychotic Symptom Rating Scales. The additionally calculated effect sizes were large, both at postassessment and at follow-up. However, reduction of distress and persecutory ideation as measured with the Green et al Paranoid Thoughts Scale did not reach significance.

Subsequently, Freeman and colleagues[43] conducted a larger scale study on individual worry-focused CBT (as described by Foster and colleagues[33]) compared with TAU. A medium-size controlled effect was found for worry and for both measures of persecutory delusions. In addition, worry was found to mediate the intervention effect on delusions, accounting for 66% of the change.

Cognitive intervention focusing on trauma

Van den Berg and colleagues[44] investigated the effect of prolonged exposure (PE), and eye movement desensitization and reprocessing (EMDR) compared with a waitlist control group. PE included in sensu and in vivo exposure. In EMDR, traumatic experiences were processed while applying eye movement as the dual-attention stimulus. Large controlled effect sizes on posttraumatic symptoms compared with the control group were reported for PE and medium-to-large controlled effect sizes for EMDR. No differences were found between intervention groups. The benefits were maintained at the 6-month follow-up. A greater decrease of paranoid thoughts at posttreatment for both interventions compared with the waitlist control group and medium-to-large controlled effect sizes were reported in an additional publication.[45] However, only the PE intervention group maintained this improvement at the 6-month follow-up. No significant effect was found on auditory hallucinations.

DISCUSSION

This review synthesized research on the effect of cognitive–behavioral interventions on depression and anxiety in patients with schizophrenia spectrum disorders. The types and formats of interventions implemented in the reviewed studies were very heterogeneous, ranging from memory training to an integrative online intervention for depression and from exposure to relaxation exercises for anxiety.

All but one of the studies focusing on depression found a positive effect on depression with medium-to-large controlled effect sizes. The only study[41] that did not find a significant controlled effect took a more conservative approach by using a fairly week intervention (an online mindfulness intervention), which was compared with a comparatively strong active control group (PMR). Five of the 6 studies on depression reported results for psychotic symptoms. Of those, only one found a significant small effect on general psychotic symptoms (ADAPT[40]) and another reported an improvement only for a specific subscale (voice-related beliefs, COMET[39]). Summing up, there seems to be substantial support suggesting a positive effect of cognitive–behavioral interventions on depression; however, not all of the interventions were sufficient in reducing psychotic symptoms.

Based on the studies available, we can only speculate on why the effects for depression did not reliably carry over to psychotic symptoms. One possibility is that the interventions were rather short and largely focused on specific aspects of depression rather than using a broader spectrum of interventions as in the state-of-the art CBT therapies for depression.[46,47] Moreover, among the 3 studies that did not find a positive effect on psychosis 2 were online based with no direct interaction between patients and therapists,[41,42] indicating that therapist contact might be a relevant factor. Another possibility is that focusing on depression only might not be sufficient to reliably reduce psychotic symptoms, and interventions need to be complemented with psychosis-specific approaches, such as working with delusional beliefs or beliefs about voices, as in CBTp.[48] To be able to draw a more definite conclusion in this regard, further and larger RCTs are needed that compare CBTp with a CBT using a comparable number of therapy sessions and format. Finally, it needs noting that, even if interventions for depression do not automatically reduce psychotic symptoms, they might nevertheless be helpful when it comes to coping with psychotic symptoms. This is indicated in the study by van der Gaag,[39] which found the cognitive interpretation of voices to change despite showing no effect of COMET on frequency or content of auditory hallucinations.

The studies focusing on anxiety all indicated positive intervention effects on anxiety or symptoms of PTSD. Controlled effect sizes ranged from small to large. Four studies assessed follow-up data and all found maintenance of the improvement. Information on results regarding psychotic symptoms were only available for 4 of the 8 studies, with 3 indicating a positive effect on at least 1 assessment scale,[33,43,44] although 1 study did not.[32] The only study that did not report an improvement was the one investigating a group-based intervention. Summing up, cognitive–behavioral interventions seem to be effective in reducing anxiety symptoms. Negative affect is known to precede and contribute to the formation and maintenance of psychotic symptoms.[11,49,50] Thus, the mechanism by which successful treatment of anxiety is likely to carry over to psychotic symptoms is by interrupting the underlying affective pathway to psychosis.[51]

Compared with depression-focused interventions, the anxiety-focused studies were somewhat more consistently able to find an improvement of psychotic symptoms. One reason for this could be that all 3 anxiety-focused interventions finding an intervention effect aimed at specific theoretically grounded mechanisms, in line with the interventionist–causal model approach,[52] with 2 studies[33,43] focusing on worry as a causal factor for paranoia[53,54] and 1 study[44] focusing on traumatic experiences.[55] The 1 study not reporting an intervention effect[32] focused on social anxiety. Although previous studies have found strong associations between social anxiety and paranoia,[56] there is no indication to date that social anxiety precedes or is causal to paranoia.[57] One can, thus, speculate that interventions that focus specifically on the causal factors, such as worry or trauma-related stress addressed in these studies, are likely to have an effect on psychotic symptoms, even if psychotic symptoms are not addressed directly, but this assumption requires further investigation.

Another aspect to consider with regard to the somewhat inconsistent results regarding psychotic symptoms is that the carry-over effect may be delayed. However, this assumption is difficult to test, with most of the studies at hand lacking long-term follow-up. Of 8 studies that conducted a follow-up,[31–33,37,38,40,43,44] only 4 reported follow-up data on psychotic symptoms. Whereas 3 studies focusing on anxiety or PTSD[33,43,44] found maintenance of the benefits at follow-up, 1 pilot study focusing on depression[38] neither found significant improvement at posttreatment nor at follow-up. A metaanalysis by Lincoln and colleagues[58] found CBTp to be superior to standard care only at follow-up regarding overall symptoms, suggesting the need of a longer time period for the CBT interventions in general to take effect on psychotic symptoms. It would, therefore, be advisable to include long-term follow-up measures in future studies.

Finally, it might also be of importance to consider the right time for a certain intervention. Because many patients already display depression- or anxiety-related symptoms at a prodromal stage,[59,60] it would be interesting to investigate whether an implementation of cognitive–behavioral interventions focusing on those target symptoms at such an early stage might be effective in reducing the risk of transiting to full psychosis.

SUMMARY

Despite the heterogeneity of the samples and interventions implemented, the majority of reviewed studies support the usefulness of using cognitive–behavioral interventions for depression- and anxiety-related problems in patients with psychosis. Whether some interventions are more suitable than others, to what extent the effects of interventions on depression and anxiety carry over to reduction of psychotic symptoms or even act as mediators of the effect on psychotic symptoms, and the precise mechanisms of action are open questions for further research.

REFERENCES

1. Buckley PF, Miller BJ, Lehrer DS, et al. Psychiatric comorbidities and schizophrenia. Schizophr Bull 2009;35(2):383–402.
2. Braga RJ, Reynolds GP, Siris SG. Anxiety comorbidity in schizophrenia. Psychiatry Res 2013;210(1):1–7.
3. Gumley A, Karatzias A, Power K, et al. Early intervention for relapse in schizophrenia: impact of cognitive behavioural therapy on negative beliefs about psychosis and self-esteem. Br J Clin Psychol 2006;45(2):247–60.
4. Lincoln TM, Lüllmann E, Rief W. Correlates and long-term consequences of poor insight in patients with schizophrenia. A systematic review. Schizophr Bull 2007; 33(6):1324–42.
5. Smith B, Fowler DG, Freeman D, et al. Emotion and psychosis: links between depression, self-esteem, negative schematic beliefs and delusions and hallucinations. Schizophr Res 2006;86(1–3):181–8.
6. Thomas N, Ribaux D, Phillips LJ. Rumination, depressive symptoms and awareness of illness in schizophrenia. Behav Cogn Psychother 2014;42(2):143–55.
7. Kleim B, Vauth R, Adam G, et al. Perceived stigma predicts low self-efficacy and poor coping in schizophrenia. J Ment Heal 2008;17(5):482–91.
8. Monti JM, Monti D. Sleep disturbance in schizophrenia. Int Rev Psychiatry 2005; 17(4):247–53.
9. Hartley S, Barrowclough C, Haddock G. Anxiety and depression in psychosis: a systematic review of associations with positive psychotic symptoms. Acta Psychiatr Scand 2013;128(5):327–46.
10. Lysaker PH, Salyers MP. Anxiety symptoms in schizophrenia spectrum disorders: associations with social function, positive and negative symptoms, hope and trauma history. Acta Psychiatr Scand 2007;116(4):290–8.
11. Garety PA, Kuipers E, Fowler D, et al. A cognitive model of the positive symptoms of psychosis. Psychol Med 2001;31(2):189–95.
12. Freeman D, Dunn G, Fowler D, et al. Current paranoid thinking in patients with delusions: the presence of cognitive-affective biases. Schizophr Bull 2013; 39(6):1281–7.

13. Fowler D, Hodgekins J, Garety P, et al. Negative cognition, depressed mood, and paranoia: a longitudinal pathway analysis using structural equation modeling. Schizophr Bull 2012;38(5):1063–73.
14. Jaya ES, Hillmann TE, Reininger KM, et al. Loneliness and psychotic symptoms: the mediating role of depression. Cognit Ther Res 2017;41(1):106–16.
15. Freeman D, Emsley R, Dunn G, et al. The stress of the street for patients with persecutory delusions: a test of the symptomatic and psychological effects of going outside into a busy urban area. Schizophr Bull 2015;41(4):971–9.
16. Freeman D, Pugh K, Antley A, et al. Virtual reality study of paranoid thinking in the general population. Br J Psychiatry 2008;192(4):258–63.
17. Startup H, Freeman D, Garety PA. Persecutory delusions and catastrophic worry in psychosis: developing the understanding of delusion distress and persistence. Behav Res Ther 2007;45(3):523–37.
18. Vorontsova N, Garety P, Freeman D. Cognitive factors maintaining persecutory delusions in psychosis: the contribution of depression. J Abnorm Psychol 2013;122(4):1121.
19. Lincoln TM, Lange J, Burau J, et al. The effect of state anxiety on paranoid ideation and jumping to conclusions. An experimental investigation. Schizophr Bull 2010;36(6):1140–8.
20. Thewissen V, Bentall RP, Oorschot M, et al. Emotions, self-esteem, and paranoid episodes: an experience sampling study. Br J Clin Psychol 2011;50(2):178–95.
21. Lincoln TM, Möbius C, Huber MT, et al. Frequency and correlates of maladaptive responses to paranoid thoughts in patients with psychosis compared to a population sample. Cogn Neuropsychiatry 2014;19(6):509–26.
22. Wüsten C, Lincoln TM. How to respond to a paranoid thought: a comparison of patients with clinically relevant delusions and healthy controls in Chile. J Nerv Ment Dis 2015;203(9):696–701.
23. Kuipers E, Garety P, Fowler D, et al. Cognitive, emotional, and social processes in psychosis: refining cognitive behavioral therapy for persistent positive symptoms. Schizophr Bull 2006;32(Suppl 1):S24–31.
24. Fowler D, Garety P, Kuipers E. Cognitive behaviour therapy for psychosis: theory and practice, vol. 25. Chichester (UK): Wiley; 1995.
25. German Association for Psychiatry, Psychotherapy and Neurology (DGPPN). S3 Praxisleitlinien in Psychiatrie Und Psychotherapie. Band 1–Behandlungsleitlinie Schizophrenie. Darmstadt (Germany): Steinkopff-Verlag; 2006.
26. National Institute for Clinical Excellence (NICE). Psychosis and schizophrenia in adults: prevention and management. NICE Guidelines. London: NICE; 2014.
27. Berry K, Haddock G. The implementation of the NICE guidelines for schizophrenia: barriers to the implementation of psychological interventions and recommendations for the future. Psychol Psychother 2008;81(4):419–36.
28. Heibach E, Brabban A, Lincoln TM. How much priority do clinicians give to cognitive behavioral therapy in the treatment of psychosis and why? Clin Psychol Sci Pract 2014;21(3):301–12.
29. Schlier B, Lincoln TM. Blinde Flecken? Der Einfluss von Stigma auf die psychotherapeutische Versorgung von Menschen mit Schizophrenie. Verhaltenstherapie 2016;26(4):279–90.
30. Moritz S, Berna F, Jaeger S, et al. The customer is always right? Subjective target symptoms and treatment preferences in patients with psychosis. Eur Arch Psychiatry Clin Neurosci 2017;267(4):335–9.

31. Chen W-C, Chu H, Lu R-B, et al. Efficacy of progressive muscle relaxation training in reducing anxiety in patients with acute schizophrenia. J Clin Nurs 2009;18(15): 2187–96.

32. Halperin S, Nathan P, Drummond P, et al. A cognitive-behavioural, group-based intervention for social anxiety in schizophrenia. Aust N Z J Psychiatry 2000;34(5): 809–13.

33. Foster C, Startup H, Potts L, et al. A randomised controlled trial of a worry intervention for individuals with persistent persecutory delusions. J Behav Ther Exp Psychiatry 2010;41(1):45–51.

34. Vancampfort D, De Hert M, Knapen J, et al. Effects of progressive muscle relaxation on state anxiety and subjective well-being in people with schizophrenia: a randomized controlled trial. Clin Rehabil 2011;25(6):567–75.

35. Georgiev A, Probst M, De Hert M, et al. Acute effects of progressive muscle relaxation on state anxiety and subjective well-being in chronic Bulgarian patients with schizophrenia. Psychiatr Danub 2012;24(4.):367–72.

36. Ricarte JJ, Hernández-Viadel JV, Latorre JM, et al. Effects of event-specific memory training on autobiographical memory retrieval and depressive symptoms in schizophrenic patients. J Behav Ther Exp Psychiatry 2012;43(Suppl 1):S12–20.

37. Kingsep P, Nathan P, Castle D. Cognitive behavioural group treatment for social anxiety in schizophrenia. Schizophr Res 2003;63(1–2):121–9.

38. Freeman D, Pugh K, Dunn G, et al. An early Phase II randomised controlled trial testing the effect on persecutory delusions of using CBT to reduce negative cognitions about the self: the potential benefits of enhancing self confidence. Schizophr Res 2014;160(1):186–92.

39. Van Der Gaag M, Van Oosterhout B, Daalman K, et al. Initial evaluation of the effects of competitive memory training (COMET) on depression in schizophrenia-spectrum patients with persistent auditory verbal hallucinations: a randomized controlled trial. Br J Clin Psychol 2012;51(2):158–71.

40. Gaudiano BA, Busch AM, Wenze SJ, et al. Acceptance-based behavior therapy for depression with psychosis: results from a pilot feasibility randomized controlled trial. J Psychiatr Pract 2015;21(5):320–33.

41. Moritz S, Cludius B, Hottenrott B, et al. Mindfulness and relaxation treatment reduce depressive symptoms in individuals with psychosis. Eur Psychiatry 2015;30(6):709–14.

42. Moritz S, Schröder J, Klein JP, et al. Effects of online intervention for depression on mood and positive symptoms in schizophrenia. Schizophr Res 2016;175(1): 216–22.

43. Freeman D, Dunn G, Startup H, et al. Effects of cognitive behaviour therapy for worry on persecutory delusions in patients with psychosis (WIT): a parallel, single-blind, randomised controlled trial with a mediation analysis. Lancet Psychiatry 2015;2(4):305–13.

44. van den Berg DPG, de Bont PAJM, van der Vleugel BM, et al. Prolonged exposure vs eye movement desensitization and reprocessing vs waiting list for posttraumatic stress disorder in patients with a psychotic disorder: a randomized clinical trial. JAMA Psychiatry 2015;72(3):259–67.

45. de Bont P, van den Berg DPG, van der Vleugel BM, et al. Prolonged exposure and EMDR for PTSD v. a PTSD waiting-list condition: effects on symptoms of psychosis, depression and social functioning in patients with chronic psychotic disorders. Psychol Med 2016;46(11):2411–21.

46. Hautzinger M, Stark W, Treiber R. Kognitive Verhaltenstherapie Bei Depressionen. Weinheim (Germany): Beltz; 2008.

47. Vittengl JR, Jarrett RB. Major depressive disorder. In: Hofmann SJ, editor. The Wiley handbook of cognitive behavioral therapy. Chicester (UK): Wiley; 2014. p. 1131–60.
48. Wykes T, Steel C, Everitt B, et al. Cognitive behavior therapy for schizophrenia: effect sizes, clinical models, and methodological rigor. Schizophr Bull 2008; 34(3):523–37.
49. Kramer I, Simons CJP, Wigman JTW, et al. Time-lagged moment-to-moment interplay between negative affect and paranoia: new insights in the affective pathway to psychosis. Schizophr Bull 2014;40(2):278–86.
50. Delespaul P, van Os J. Determinants of occurrence and recovery from hallucinations in daily life. Soc Psychiatry Psychiatr Epidemiol 2002;37(3):97–104.
51. Myin-Germeys I, van Os J. Stress-reactivity in psychosis: evidence for an affective pathway to psychosis. Clin Psychol Rev 2007;27(4):409–24.
52. Kendler KS, Campbell J. Interventionist causal models in psychiatry: repositioning the mind–body problem. Psychol Med 2009;39(6):881–7.
53. Freeman D, Freeman J. Paranoia: the 21st century fear. Oxford (England): Oxford University Press; 2008.
54. Freeman D, Stahl D, McManus S, et al. Insomnia, worry, anxiety and depression as predictors of the occurrence and persistence of paranoid thinking. Soc Psychiatry Psychiatr Epidemiol 2012;47(8):1195–203.
55. Sareen J, Cox BJ, Goodwin RD, et al. Co-occurrence of posttraumatic stress disorder with positive psychotic symptoms in a nationally representative sample. J Trauma Stress 2005;18(4):313–22.
56. Gilbert P, Boxall M, Cheung M, et al. The relation of paranoid ideation and social anxiety in a mixed clinical population. Clin Psychol Psychother 2005;12(2): 124–33.
57. Rietdijk J, Van Os J, de Graaf R, et al. Are social phobia and paranoia related, and which comes first? Psychosis 2009;1(1):29–38.
58. Lincoln TM, Suttner C, Nestoriuc Y. Wirksamkeit kognitiver Interventionen für Schizophrenie: Eine Meta-Analyse. Psychol Rundsch 2008;59(4):217–32.
59. Häfner H, Maurer K, An der Heiden W. ABC Schizophrenia study: an overview of results since 1996. Soc Psychiatry Psychiatr Epidemiol 2013;48(7):1021–31.
60. van der Gaag M, Nieman DH, Rietdijk J, et al. Cognitive behavioral therapy for subjects at ultrahigh risk for developing psychosis: a randomized controlled clinical trial. Schizophr Bull 2012;38(6):1180–8.

Cognitive Behavioral Therapy for Anxiety and Depression in Children and Adolescents

Ella L. Oar, PhD[a],*, Carly Johnco, PhD[a], Thomas H. Ollendick, PhD[b]

KEYWORDS

- Anxiety • Depression • Child • Adolescent • Cognitive therapy • Behavior therapy

KEY POINTS

- Anxiety and depression are highly prevalent in youth.
- Assessments for youth should ideally be multimethod and multi-informant.
- Cognitive behavioral therapy (CBT) has received strong empirical support for the treatment of anxiety and depression in youth.
- Latest research in the field is focused on innovative approaches to enhance CBT, the personalization of treatment, and increasing access to treatment using technology.

Anxiety and depressive disorders are the most common mental health conditions affecting children and adolescents.[1] Anxiety and depression are commonly comorbid in youth, overlapping in symptoms, cause, and sequelae.[2] However, despite their common cooccurrence, these disorders are also distinct. This review summarizes the most up-to-date information on the phenomenology, assessment, and treatment of anxiety and depressive disorders in children and adolescents, as well as highlights some of the more recent and novel developments in treatment approaches for these disorders.

PHENOMENOLOGY OF ANXIETY DISORDERS IN YOUTH

Anxiety disorders are the most common mental health problem during childhood and adolescence, with lifetime prevalence rates ranging from 9% to 30%.[1,3] Many anxiety

The authors have nothing to disclose.
[a] Centre for Emotional Health, Department of Psychology, Macquarie University, Level 1 Australian Hearing Hub, 16 University Avenue, Sydney, New South Wales 2109, Australia;
[b] Child Study Center, Virginia Polytechnic Institute and State University, Suite 207, 460 Turner Street, Blacksburg, VA 24060, USA
* Corresponding author.
E-mail address: ella.oar@mq.edu.au

Psychiatr Clin N Am 40 (2017) 661–674
http://dx.doi.org/10.1016/j.psc.2017.08.002
0193-953X/17/© 2017 Elsevier Inc. All rights reserved.

psych.theclinics.com

disorders have their onset during childhood, with separation anxiety disorder (SAD) and specific phobias usually occurring before age 10, social anxiety disorder (SoAD) tending to emerge during late childhood and early adolescence, and panic disorder and agoraphobia usually having an age of onset during late adolescence or early adulthood.[3,4] There is less consistent evidence for the age of onset of generalized anxiety disorder (GAD). Anxiety disorders are more common in girls and women, with the gender difference beginning in childhood and showing an increase over development.[4] Anxiety disorders have a deleterious short- and long-term impact on youth. In the short term, children with anxiety disorders tend to show poorer academic performance and impairments in social and family functioning.[5] Contrary to common beliefs that children will "grow out" of their anxiety, untreated childhood anxiety is often unremitting into adulthood and increases the risk of developing other mental health problems (eg, depressive and substance use disorders).[6]

PHENOMENOLOGY OF DEPRESSIVE DISORDERS IN YOUTH

In children, depressive disorders can also be characterized by extreme irritability rather than sad mood or anhedonia.[7] With the typical age on onset between 11 and 14 years,[8] prevalence rates for mood disorders in children are relatively low (<1%),[9] although this increases substantially during adolescence, with prevalence estimates ranging up to 14%.[1] This increase is often attributed to pubertal and social changes during adolescence.[10] Mood disorders in youth are associated with serious impairments in social, academic, and occupational functioning[11,12] as well as smoking and alcohol abuse.[13] In addition, adolescents with major depression are 27 times more likely to die by suicide.[14] During childhood, there are either no gender differences in mood disorders or slightly higher rates in boys; however, this gender distribution changes in adolescence to an increased prevalence (around 2:1) among girls.[15] Although most adolescents recover from their initial depressive episode, 50% to 70% relapse within 5 years.[16,17] Similar to anxiety, depression in childhood and adolescence is associated with an increased risk of adult anxiety, substance-use disorders, suicidal behavior, and unemployment.[18,19]

EVIDENCED-BASED ASSESSMENT

Anxiety and depression symptoms both lie on a continuum of severity. Accurate assessment is the foundation upon which treatment planning and monitoring is built, and current recommendations are that youth are screened for symptoms of anxiety, depression, and functional impairment, and that a comprehensive diagnostic evaluation be undertaken if symptoms are present.[20] In youth, it is important to not only accurately diagnose anxiety and depression but also detect the presence of subsyndromal symptoms, because youth with subsyndromal symptoms are at high risk of developing full-threshold disorders over time.[21]

There are 2 main methods used to assess anxiety and depression in youth: clinician-administered instruments and parent- and youth-report questionnaire-based measures of symptoms and symptom severity. Although a detailed description of measures is beyond the scope of this review, the most commonly used measures are briefly summarized in later discussion.

Clinician-Administered Diagnostic Interviews and Symptom Measures

Clinician-administered diagnostic interviews are the most comprehensive, reliable, and valid method to determine diagnostic status for youth with these disorders. Diagnosing anxiety and mood disorders in youth requires knowledge of normal child development to facilitate differentiation of transient fears and mood lability. The most commonly used measures are the Anxiety Disorders Interview Schedule for Diagnostic and Statistical Manual of Mental Disorders (DSM-IV) (4th edition), Child and Parent version (ADIS-IV-C/P),[22] Kiddie Schedule for Affective Disorders and Schizophrenia (K-SADS-P/L),[23] the National Institute of Mental Health (NIMH) Diagnostic Interview Schedule for Children (DISC),[24] and the Mini International Neuropsychiatric Interview for Children and Adolescents (MINI-KID).[25] These interviews are administered to the young person and their parent (usually separately), with a final diagnosis determined by the clinician based on all available information.

The ADIS-C/P is one of the most widely used semistructured measures of anxiety and depression and assesses the presence of current diagnoses in youth. Questions follow diagnostic criteria and include prompts for anxiety-provoking situations and topics of worry, with a visual prompt (a "thermometer") aiding youth and parents to rate the severity of fear, worry, physiologic symptoms, and interference. The ADIS differs from other diagnostic interviews in that it provides information not only relating to the presence of a diagnosis but also to the severity of each disorder on a 0 to 8 scale, with severity ratings ≥ 4 indicative of clinical diagnoses.

The K-SADS-PL is another semistructured interview that assesses both present and lifetime episodes of psychopathology in children and adolescents. Administration requires clinical expertise, with the interviewer asking a range of semistructured questions based around a theme to determine whether the child meets the diagnostic criteria.

The DISC is a highly structured interview developed by the NIMH designed to be used by lay interviewers. Questions use verbatim prompts and structured response options. This interview differs from the ADIS and K-SADS in that diagnostic status is determined by a computer algorithm.

The MINI-KID is a more recently developed measure of child and adolescent psychopathology and is intended as a comprehensive but brief structured diagnostic interview. This measure takes approximately half an hour to administer, making it significantly faster to administer than other interviews.

The 2 most prominent clinician-administered measures of anxiety and depression *severity* (as opposed to diagnostic status) for children and adolescents are the Children's Depression Rating Scale-Revised[26] and the Pediatric Anxiety Rating Scale.[27]

Parent and Child-Report Measures

There are several available measures for assessing the severity of anxiety and depression symptoms in children and adolescents. Most of these measures include child- and parent-report versions and are useful for assessing the presence and severity of a range of symptoms. Many of these scales include subscales that align with specific diagnostic categories. The most commonly used measures of pediatric anxiety and depression symptoms are summarized in **Table 1**.

EVIDENCE-BASED TREATMENT

Cognitive behavioral therapy (CBT) is efficacious for treating anxiety and depression in youth. It addresses the maladaptive thoughts and behaviors that underlie these disorders. CBT incorporates a range of techniques to enhance children and adolescent's awareness and understanding of emotions, increase cognitive flexibility, challenge anxious or negative appraisals, increase behavioral activation, and decrease escape and avoidance.[44] Core CBT strategies for anxious and depressed youth

Table 1
Questionnaire measures of anxiety and depression symptoms in youth

Measure	Domain	Number of Items	Scores and Subscales
Spence Children's Anxiety Scale (SCAS)[28]	Anxiety	Child: 44 items (38 reflective of anxiety and 6 filler items) Parent: 38 items	Total score, separation anxiety, social phobia, obsessive compulsive, panic/agoraphobia, physical injury fears, and generalized anxiety
Multidimensional Anxiety Scale for Children–2nd Edition (MASC-2)[29]	Anxiety	Child: 50 items Parent: 50 items	Total score; separation anxiety/phobias; GAD Index Social anxiety total; humiliation/rejection; performance fears; obsessions & compulsions; physical symptoms; harm avoidance; inconsistency index (response style)
Screen for Child Anxiety-related Emotional Disorders (SCARED)[30]	Anxiety	Child: 41 items Parent: 41 items	Total score; GAD, SAD, SoAD, panic disorder, and school phobia
Fear Survey Schedule for Children–Revised (FSSC-R)[31]	Anxiety	Child: 80 items Parent: 80 items	Failure and criticism; the unknown; minor injury and small animals; danger and death; medical fears
Patient-Reported Outcomes Measurement Information System (PROMIS)– Pediatric Anxiety Symptoms scale[32]	Anxiety	Child: 8 items (or 4- and 6-item short form) Parent: 8 items (or 4- and 6-item short form)	Total
Revised Children's Manifest Anxiety Scale–2nd Edition (RCMAS-2)[33]	Anxiety	Child: 49 items (or 10-item short form) Parent: N/A	Total; physiologic anxiety, worry; social anxiety, defensiveness subscale (response style), inconsistent responding index (response style)
State-Trait Anxiety Inventory for Children–Trait version (STAI-C)[34]	Anxiety	Child: 20 items Parent: 26 items	Trait anxiety (state anxiety version also available)
Revised Child Anxiety and Depression Scale (RCADS)[35]	Anxiety and depression	Child: 47 items Parent: 47 items	Total score, anxiety total, separation anxiety, social phobia, obsessive compulsive, panic/agoraphobia, generalized anxiety, major depression

(continued on next page)

Table 1 (continued)			
Measure	**Domain**	**Number of Items**	**Scores and Subscales**
Short Mood Feeling Questionnaire[36]	Depression	Child: 13 items Parent: 13 items	Total
Children's Depression Inventory–2nd edition (CDI-2)[37]	Depression	Child: 28 items (or 12-item short form) Parent: 17 items	Total score, emotional problems, functional problems, negative mood Negative self-esteem Ineffectiveness, interpersonal problems
Reynolds Child Depression Scale–2nd edition (RCDS-2)[38]	Depression	Child: 30 items (or 11-item short form) Parent: N/A	Total
Reynolds Adolescent Depression scale–2nd edition (RADS-2)[39]	Depression	Child: 30 items Parent: N/A	Total; dysphoric mood, anhedonia/negative affect, negative self-evaluation, and somatic complaints
Center for Epidemiological Studies Depression Scale for Children (CES-DC)[40]	Depression	Child: 20 items Parent: N/A	Total score
Beck Depression Inventory for Youth[41]	Depression	Child: 20 items Parent: N/A	Total score
Depression Self-Rating Scale (DSRS)[42]	Depression	Child: 18 items Parent: N/A	Total
PROMIS Pediatric Depressive Symptoms Scale[32]	Depression	Child: 8 items (or 4- and 6-item short form) Parent: 8 items (or 4- and 6-item short form)	Total
Suicidal Ideation Questionnaire–Junior (SIQ-Jr)[43]	Suicidal ideation	Child: 15 items Parent: N/A	Total

Abbreviation: N/A, not applicable.

typically include psychoeducation, cognitive restructuring, exposure, and behavioral activation.

Treatment of Anxiety Disorders in Youth

To date, most controlled trials for anxious children and adolescents have evaluated the effectiveness of broad-based CBT protocols, designed to treat a range of diagnoses (eg, SAD, GAD, and SoAD) by targeting the shared underlying features. Broad-based protocols have been delivered individually, in group settings, and via the Internet, and typically involve 9 to 20 sessions.[45] The first large randomized controlled trial (RCT) for anxious youth was conducted in the 1990s and examined the relative efficacy of "Coping Cat," a 16-session broad-based CBT program compared with a wait-list control.[46] There are now several manualized broad-based CBT protocols available including the "Coping Cat program,"[47] "Cool Kids program,"[48] and the "Take ACTION program."[49]

Support has also been found for disorder-specific treatments for GAD,[50] SAD,[51] SoAD,[52] and panic disorder.[53] With the exception of the one-session treatment (OST) approach for youth with specific phobias, these targeted approaches have not been as extensively evaluated as broad-based treatments. OST for phobic youth has a strong evidence base with 3 large RCTs and 7 smaller trials supporting its effectiveness[54] compared with wait-list[55] and active control conditions.[56,57]

The largest RCT for anxious youth to date, and the only trial to evaluate the relative efficacy of CBT compared with pharmacologic treatment, is the Child/Adolescent Anxiety Multimodal Study. This trial randomly assigned 488 youth (7–17 years) to CBT (Coping Cat), sertraline (SRT), combined CBT and SRT (COMB), or placebo pill (PBO). At posttreatment, COMB outperformed CBT and SRT on primary outcomes measures and remission rates.[58,59] All active treatments (COMB, CBT, SRT) led to significantly better outcomes compared with PBO.

Several systematic reviews and meta-analyses have been conducted in order to summarize the extant child anxiety treatment literature.[45,60] A meta-analysis of 41 studies (1806 participants)[45] concluded that CBT was more effective than wait-list control conditions, with remission rates of 59%, compared with 16% for wait-list control conditions.[45] Although there was some evidence for the superiority CBT in comparison to active controls, the results were nonsignificant and limited because of the small number of published studies. Moreover, outcomes did not differ between individual, group, and parent/family-based CBT. The most recent review of evidence-based treatments for child anxiety[60] from 111 studies concluded that 6 variants of CBT (CBT, exposure, modeling, CBT with parents, education, and CBT combination with medication) reached *well-established* status for treatment of anxious youth.

Treatment of Depressive Disorders in Youth

Three psychological therapies have received empiric support for the treatment of child and adolescent depression: CBT, Interpersonal Psychotherapy (IPT), and family therapy; however, of those, CBT is the most well established.[61] Typically, CBT for depressed youth ranges from 5 to 16 sessions. It too has been delivered in individual and group formats and via Internet delivery. The Coping with Depression for Adolescents program (Clarke GN, Lewinsohn PM, unpublished data, 1986), the ACTION program,[62] and the Primary and Secondary Control Enhancement Training[63] are all widely used evidence-based manualized CBT programs.

The largest treatment trial to date for depressed youth was the multisite Treatment for Adolescents with Depression Study.[64] Adolescents (N = 439) aged 12 to 17 with primary Major Depressive Disorder diagnoses were randomly assigned to CBT (15 sessions), fluoxetine (FLX), COMB, or PBO for 12 weeks. At posttreatment, COMB was associated with greater improvements than FLX and CBT alone on primary outcomes measures: FLX was superior to CBT; and, CBT was no more beneficial than PBO. The disappointing findings in relation to CBT received considerable attention with some suggestion that the type of CBT (eg, limited number of sessions with many and varied treatment components) and the manner in which CBT was implemented may have led to the poorer outcomes.[65] At long-term follow-up, however, CBT outcomes were comparable to FLX and COMB. In addition, although rates of suicidal events decreased over the course of therapy, this was less so for FLX in comparison to COMB and CBT.[66]

A recent review of psychosocial treatments for depression[61] identified 42 published RCTs. Poorer evidence was found for child CBT (<13 years) relative to adolescent CBT

(13–24 years), although only 7 RCTs evaluated the efficacy of CBT for depressed children. Within child samples, CBT was found to be superior to wait-list control conditions; however, it was not consistently found to be superior to other active controls or alternate evidence-based treatments. Thus, given these mixed findings, CBT for depressed children only met *possibly efficacious* status. In comparison, 27 RCTs evaluated the efficacy of CBT in adolescent samples. Across studies, CBT was superior to wait-list control conditions, and most studies found that CBT outperformed active controls and alternate treatments. Thus, for adolescents, CBT is considered a *well-established* treatment. IPT was similarly found to meet *well-established* criteria for depressed adolescents; however, only 6 RCTs have been conducted.

Transdiagnostic Approaches to Treatment in Youth

Recent years have seen the emergence of transdiagnostic CBT protocols for youth. These protocols are designed to treat both anxiety and depression together and were developed because of (1) the high comorbidity between the disorders (up to 75%),[67] (2) shared developmental pathways, and (3) research indicating that comorbidity between the disorders may lead to a poorer treatment response to specific, single-disorder treatments.[68,69] Drawing upon a unified theoretic model,[70] transdiagnostic treatments aim to address the common mechanisms and maintaining factors underlying both anxiety and depression to maximize treatment outcome and durability, differentiating it from eclectic treatment approaches.[71] Two controlled trials have recently been published that provide support for the approach in youth.[44,70,72,73]

A preliminary RCT with 35 youth (12–14 years) who met criteria for current clinical or subclinical primary anxiety or unipolar depressive disorder examined the relative efficacy of a group-based transdiagnostic behavioral activation treatment (GBAT) to a wait-list control group.[73] GBAT consisted of psychoeducation, problem solving, exposure, and behavioral activation and was delivered in a school setting over 10 sessions. Compared with the wait-list control group, those in the GBAT showed improved posttreatment outcomes in impairment and remission rates of secondary diagnoses.[73] Overall, remission rates for GBAT were 57% for primary diagnosis and 70% for secondary diagnosis, compared with 28% and 10%, respectively, in the wait-list condition. No group differences were observed on self-report measures.

The second transdiagnostic trial was conducted with 51 adolescents (12–17 years) with a primary diagnosis of an anxiety disorder or unipolar depression.[44] Participants were randomly assigned to a unified treatment protocol for emotional disorders in adolescents (UP-A) or a wait-list control. UP-A involved 8 to 21 sessions with all youth completing 5 core treatment modules (affective education, emotional awareness, cognitive flexibility, exposure/behavioral activation, and relapse prevention) and supplementary modules (building motivation, suicidality and managing intense emotions, and parent management) as indicated. At posttreatment, UP-A was associated with superior improvement across all outcome measures in comparison to the wait-list control.[44] Although transdiagnostic treatments require further evaluation, particularly in relation to their benefit above and beyond traditional single-disorder treatments, these trials provide exciting initial support.

RECENT DEVELOPMENTS IN TREATMENTS FOR YOUTH ANXIETY AND DEPRESSION

There have been several recent developments in the child anxiety and depression fields that have focused on novel approaches to enhancing CBT: the personalization of treatment to maximize outcome, and improving treatment accessibility.[74] Although CBT is effective for the most anxious and depressed youth, a significant proportion fails to respond to treatment and continue to experience clinically significant symptoms.[45,75] Current research in both the child anxiety and the depression fields has explored the effectiveness of cognitive bias modification (CBM) training as a stand-alone treatment or augmentation to standard CBT. These treatments are proposed to work by the modifying attentional (CBM-A) and interpretation (CBM-I) biases that underlie anxiety and depression.[76] CBM-A interventions typically involve youth learning to direct their attention away from negative/threat stimuli (eg, pictures or words) toward neutral or positive stimuli. CBM-I involves teaching youth to interpret ambiguous stimuli (eg, paragraphs or sentences) less negatively.[77] The first meta-analysis of 23 RCTs of CBM for children and adolescents was recently conducted.[76] Overall, only small effects were found in favor of the CBM interventions. For anxiety, the number needed to treat (NNT) was 10.42, whereas for depression it was 166.67.[76] The investigators stated that the quality of RCTs included in the meta-analysis was less than ideal and that most studies did not include the necessary information to complete a quality assessment. They called for large-scale RCTs, in clinical samples of youth, using standardized treatment protocols, to provide more conclusive evidence regarding the benefits of CBM-A/I approaches for youth.

Another avenue of research currently being explored is the personalization of CBT approaches. Existing CBT protocols are highly routinized, with children typically completing the same session-by-session treatment sequence and covering the same content. However, as noted previously, not all children respond to these standard treatments. Exciting new work has used results from treatment predictor studies to highlight poor prognostic characteristics and to generate algorithms or indices to identify youth who present with characteristics related to poorer treatment response.[78] Work continues with these at-risk youth to understand whether enhanced or personalized treatment approaches may help to improve outcome. For example, as previously discussed, cooccurring anxiety and depression have been found to be associated with a poorer response to treatment,[68,69] which has led to the development of innovative transdiagnostic treatment approaches. Another example of tailoring interventions involves the use of modular-based treatment approaches. These approaches take treatment strategies from established treatments and incorporate them into stand-alone modules.[78] These modules are then combined through the use of decision-making flowcharts to tailor treatment of the individual. The Modular Approach to Therapy for Children (MATCH)[79] was one of the first modular treatments for youth. This program includes a collection of modules that target symptoms of anxiety, depression, trauma, and disruptive behavior. Based on the child's primary presenting problem, 1 of 4 (eg, anxiety, depression, trauma, and disruptive behavior) flow decision charts are selected. The clinician then completes, with the child, the core default modules relating to the selected disorder.[79] As treatment progresses, additional modules may be included based on the child's unique clinical presentation (eg, comorbidity or treatment interfering variables) or core modules repeated if necessary. The efficacy of MATCH has been evaluated in a large RCT ($N = 174$) in comparison to usual care and standard evidenced-based treatment (eg, Coping Cat; Primary and Secondary Control Enhancement Training; and Defiant Children) within the community.[80] Those in the MATCH condition had fewer diagnoses at posttreatment and showed faster rates of improvement in comparison to usual care.[80] However, there were no significant differences between MATCH and standard evidence-based care in relation to the number of diagnoses at posttreatment or change trajectories.[80] Standard treatment did not differ from usual care in relation to number of diagnoses at posttreatment. Overall, this study provided preliminary support for the additional benefit of modular-based treatment approaches in comparison to standard evidence-based approaches.

Despite its demonstrated effectiveness, only a small proportion of youth receive CBT for the treatment of anxiety or depression. In an effort to increase accessibility to evidence-based treatments the last decade has seen the emergence of Internet and computerized approaches to delivering CBT. A recent review of 13 RCTs[81] of computer-, Internet-, and mobile phone–delivered CBT interventions for children and adolescents included 7 trials targeting anxiety, 4 targeting depression, and 2 transdiagnostic trials. Overall, moderate to large effects (g = 0.72; NNT = 2.56) were found in favor of CBT. Another recent review[82] explored the efficacy of Internet-delivered CBT for children and adolescents with psychiatric and somatic conditions. Twenty-five trials were identified, with most conducted in samples of anxious youth (n = 6 in total; n = 5 RCTs) and only one trial in depressed youth. CBT was found to show moderate to large effects (g = .62) in comparison to wait-list controls. Overall, Internet and computerized treatments appear to offer a promising alternative to traditional face-to-face delivery and have additional benefits in terms of accessibility and affordability of evidence-based treatments.

SUMMARY

Anxiety and depressive disorders are highly prevalent in children and adolescents.[1] These disorders commonly cooccur in youth and overlap in terms of their symptoms, cause, and sequelae.[2] Clinician-administered instruments, such as diagnostic and clinician-administered interviews and parent- and youth-report questionnaires, are the most commonly used methods to assess for anxiety and depression in youth. Ideally, assessments for youth should use multiple methods (eg, diagnostic interview and questionnaires) and involve multiple informants (eg, the child, parents, and teachers). CBT is considered a first-line treatment of anxiety and depression in youth and possesses a strong evidence base. It incorporates psychoeducation, cognitive restructuring, exposure, and behavioral activation. The latest research in the field has focused on innovative approaches to enhance CBT, and the personalization of treatment.[74] To address difficulties in accessing treatment of youth, researchers have begun to evaluate the efficacy of computer-, Internet-, and mobile phone–delivered CBT, with promising outcomes to date. Over the past 20 years, considerable progress has been made in treating anxiety and depression using CBT in youth; however, with less than optimal remission rates, more is needed to improve outcomes for youth who fail to respond to the current best treatments.

REFERENCES

1. Merikangas KR, He JP, Burstein M, et al. Lifetime prevalence of mental disorders in US adolescents: results from the National Comorbidity Study-Adolescent Supplement (NCS-A). J Am Acad Child Adolesc Psychiatry 2010;49(10):980–9.

2. Garber J, Weersing VR. Comorbidity of anxiety and depression in youth: implications for treatment and prevention. Clin Psychol (New York) 2010;17(4):293–306.

3. Beesdo K, Knappe S, Pine DS. Anxiety and anxiety disorders in children and adolescents: developmental issues and implications for DSM-V. Psychiatr Clin North Am 2009;32(3):483–524.

4. Rapee RM, Schniering CA, Hudson JL. Anxiety disorders during childhood and adolescence: origins and treatment. Annu Rev Clin Psychol 2009;5(1):311–41.

5. Essau CA, Conradt J, Petermann F. Frequency, comorbidity, and psychosocial impairment of anxiety disorders in german adolescents. J Anxiety Disord 2000; 14(3):263–79.
6. Woodward LJ, Fergusson DM. Life course outcomes of young people with anxiety disorders in adolescence. J Am Acad Child Adolesc Psychiatry 2001;40(9): 1086–93.
7. American Psychiatric Association. Diagnostic and statistical manual of mental disorders. 5th edition. Arlington (VA): American Psychiatric Publishing; 2013.
8. Lewinsohn PM, Rohde P, Seeley JR, et al. Age-cohort changes in the lifetime occurrence of depression and other mental disorders. J Abnorm Psychol 1993; 102(1):110–20.
9. Kessler RC, Avenevoli S, Ries Merikangas K. Mood disorders in children and adolescents: an epidemiologic perspective. Biol Psychiatry 2001;49(12):1002–14.
10. Cyranowski JM, Frank E, Young E, et al. Adolescent onset of the gender difference in lifetime rates of major depression: a theoretical model. Arch Gen Psychiatry 2000;57(1):21–7.
11. Fletcher JM. Adolescent depression: diagnosis, treatment, and educational attainment. Health Econ 2008;17(11):1215–35.
12. Rao U, Chen LA. Characteristics, correlates, and outcomes of childhood and adolescent depressive disorders. Dialogues Clin Neurosci 2009;11(1):45–62.
13. Haarasilta LM, Marttunen MJ, Kaprio JA, et al. Correlates of depression in a representative nationwide sample of adolescents (15-19 years) and young adults (20-24 years). Eur J Public Health 2004;14(3):280–5.
14. Brent DA, Perper JA, Moritz G, et al. Psychiatric risk factors for adolescent suicide: a case-control study. J Am Acad Child Adolesc Psychiatry 1993;32(3): 521–9.
15. Cohen P, Cohen J, Kasen S, et al. An epidemiological study of disorders in late childhood and adolescence–I. Age- and gender-specific prevalence. J Child Psychol Psychiatry 1993;34(6):851–67.
16. Dunn V, Goodyer IM. Longitudinal investigation into childhood and adolescence onset depression: psychiatric outcome in early adulthood. Br J Psychiatry 2006; 188:216–22.
17. Lewinsohn PM, Rohde P, Seeley JR, et al. Natural course of adolescent major depressive disorder in a community sample: predictors of recurrence in young adults. Am J Psychiatry 2000;157(10):1584–91.
18. Kim-Cohen J, Caspi A, Moffitt TE, et al. Prior juvenile diagnoses in adults with mental disorder: developmental follow-back of a prospective-longitudinal cohort. Arch Gen Psychiatry 2003;60(7):709–17.
19. Thapar A, Collishaw S, Pine DS, et al. Depression in adolescence. Lancet 2012; 379(9820):1056–67.
20. Connolly SD, Bernstein GA. Practice parameter for the assessment and treatment of children and adolescents with anxiety disorders. J Am Acad Child Adolesc Psychiatry 2007;46(2):267–83.
21. Fergusson DM, Horwood LJ, Ridder EM, et al. Subthreshold depression in adolescence and mental health outcomes in adulthood. Arch Gen Psychiatry 2005;62(1):66–72.
22. Silverman WK, Albano AM. The anxiety disorders interview schedule for DSM-IV-child and parent versions. San Antonio (TX): Graywinds Publications; 1996.
23. Kaufman J, Birmaher B, Brent D, et al. Schedule for affective disorders and schizophrenia for school-age children-present and lifetime version (K-SADS-PL): initial reliability and validity data. J Am Acad Child Adolesc Psychiatry 1997;36(7):980–8.

24. Shaffer D, Fisher P, Lucas CP, et al. NIMH Diagnostic Interview Schedule for Children Version IV (NIMH DISC-IV): description, differences from previous versions, and reliability of some common diagnoses. J Am Acad Child Adolesc Psychiatry 2000;39(1):28–38.

25. Sheehan DV, Sheehan KH, Shytle RD, et al. Reliability and validity of the Mini International Neuropsychiatric Interview for Children and Adolescents (MINI-KID). J Clin Psychiatry 2010;71(3):313–26.

26. Poznanski EO, Mokros HB. Children's depression rating scale revised manual. Los Angeles (CA): Western Psychological Services; 1996.

27. The Research Units On Pediatric Psychopharmacology Anxiety Study Group (RUPP). The Pediatric Anxiety Rating Scale (PARS): development and psychometric properties. J Am Acad Child Adolesc Psychiatry 2002;41(9):1061–9.

28. Spence SH. A measure of anxiety symptoms among children. Behav Res Ther 1998;36(5):545–66.

29. March JS. The multidimensional anxiety scale for children - 2nd edition (MASC-2). Toronto: MultiHealth Systems; 2012.

30. Birmaher B, Khetarpal S, Brent D, et al. The screen for child anxiety related emotional disorders (SCARED): scale construction and psychometric characteristics. J Am Acad Child Adolesc Psychiatry 1997;36(4):545–53.

31. Ollendick TH. Reliability and validity of the revised fear survey schedule for children (FSSC-R). Behav Res Ther 1983;21(6):685–92.

32. Irwin DE, Stucky B, Langer MM, et al. An item response analysis of the pediatric PROMIS anxiety and depressive symptoms scales. Qual Life Res 2010;19(4):595–607.

33. Reynolds CR, Richmond BO. The revised children's manifest anxiety scale, second edition (RCMAS-2). Los Angeles (CA): Western Psychological Services; 2008.

34. Spielberger CD. Manual for the state-trait anxiety inventory for children. Palo Alto (CA): Consulting Psychologists Press; 1973.

35. Chorpita BF, Yim L, Moffitt C, et al. Assessment of symptoms of DSM-IV anxiety and depression in children: a revised child anxiety and depression scale. Behav Res Ther 2000;38(8):835–55.

36. Angold A, Costello EJ, Messer SC, et al. Development of a short questionnaire for use in epidemiological studies of depression in children and adolescents. Int J Methods Psychiatr Res 1995;5:237–49.

37. Kovacs M. Children's depression inventory 2 (CDI 2). 2nd edition. North Tonawanda (NY): Multi-Health Systems Inc; 2011.

38. Reynolds WM. Reynolds child depression scale. 2nd edition. Lutz (FL): Psychological Assessment Resources; 2002.

39. Reynolds WM. Reynolds adolescent depression scale. 2nd edition. Lutz (FL): Psychological Assessment Resources; 2002.

40. Weissman MM, Orvaschel H, Padian N. Children's symptom and social functioning self-report scales: comparison of mothers' and children's reports. J Nerv Ment Dis 1980;168(12):736–40.

41. Beck JS, Beck AT, Jolly JB. Beck youth inventories. San Antonio (TX): Psychological Corporation; 2001.

42. Birleson P. The validity of depressive disorder in childhood and the development of a self-rating scale: a research report. J Child Psychol Psychiatry 1981;22(1):73–88.

43. Reynolds WM. Suicidal ideation questionnaire: professional manual. Odessa (FL): Psychological Assessment Resources; 1988.

44. Ehrenreich-May J, Rosenfield D, Queen AH, et al. An initial waitlist-controlled trial of the unified protocol for the treatment of emotional disorders in adolescents. J Anxiety Disord 2017;46:46–55.
45. James AC, James G, Cowdrey FA, et al. Cognitive behavioural therapy for anxiety disorders in children and adolescents. Cochrane Database Syst Rev 2013;(6):CD004690.
46. Kendall PC. Treating anxiety disorders in children: results of a randomized clinical trial. J Consult Clin Psychol 1994;62(1):100–10.
47. Kendall PC, Hedtke KA. Cognitive-behavioral therapy for anxious children: therapist manual. 3rd edition. Admore (PA): Workbook Publishing; 2006.
48. Rapee RM, Lyneham HJ, Schniering CA, et al. Cool kids: child & adolescent anxiety program. Sydney (Australia): Centre for Emotional Health, Macquarie University; 2006.
49. Waters AM, Groth T. Take action practitioner guidebook. Samford Valley (Queensland): Australian Academic Press; 2016.
50. Holmes MC, Donovan CL, Farrell LJ, et al. The efficacy of a group-based, disorder-specific treatment program for childhood GAD – a randomized controlled trial. Behav Res Ther 2014;61:122–35.
51. Schneider S, Blatter-Meunier J, Herren C, et al. Disorder-specific cognitive-behavioral therapy for separation anxiety disorder in young children: a randomized waiting-list-controlled trial. Psychother Psychosom 2011;80(4):206–15.
52. Beidel DC, Turner SM, Morris TL. Behavioral treatment of childhood social phobia. J Consult Clin Psychol 2000;68(6):1072–80.
53. Gallo KP, Chan PT, Buzzella BA, et al. The impact of an 8-day intensive treatment for adolescent panic disorder and agoraphobia on comorbid diagnoses. Behav Ther 2012;43(1):153–9.
54. Oar EL, Farrell LJ, Byrne SP, et al. Specific phobia. In: Flessner CA, Piacentini J, editors. Clinical handbook of psychological disorders in children and adolescents: a step-by-step treatment manual. New York: The Guilford Press; 2017. p. 169–203.
55. Öst LG, Svensson L, Hellstrom K, et al. One-session treatment of specific phobias in youths: a randomized clinical trial. J Consult Clin Psychol 2001;69(5):814–24.
56. Ollendick TH, Öst LG, Reuterskiold L, et al. One-session treatment of specific phobias in youth: a randomized clinical trial in the United States and Sweden. J Consult Clin Psychol 2009;77(3):504–16.
57. Ollendick TH, Halldorsdottir T, Fraire MG, et al. Specific phobias in youth: a randomized controlled trial comparing one-session treatment to a parent-augmented one-session treatment. Behav Ther 2015;46:141–55.
58. Ginsburg GS, Sakolsky D, Piacentini JC, et al. Remission after acute treatment in children and adolescents with anxiety disorders: findings from the CAMS. J Consult Clin Psychol 2011;79(6):806–13.
59. Walkup JT, Albano AM, Piacentini J, et al. Cognitive behavioral therapy, sertraline, or a combination in childhood anxiety. N Engl J Med 2008;359(26):2753–66.
60. Higa-McMillan CK, Francis SE, Rith-Najarian L, et al. Evidence base update: 50 years of research on treatment for child and adolescent anxiety. J Clin Child Adolesc Psychol 2016;45(2):91–113.
61. Weersing VR, Jeffreys M, Do MCT, et al. Evidence base update of psychosocial treatments for child and adolescent depression. J Clin Child Adolesc Psychol 2017;46(1):11–43.
62. Stark KD, Streusand W, Krumholz LS, et al. Cognitive-behavioral therapy for depression: the ACTION treatment program for girls. In: Weisz JR, Kazdin AE,

editors. Evidence-based psychotherapies for children and adolescents. 2nd edition. New York: Guilford Press; 2010. p. 93–109.

63. Weisz JR, Southam-Gerow MA, Gordis EB, et al. Cognitive–behavioral therapy versus usual clinical care for youth depression: an initial test of transportability to community clinics and clinicians. J Consult Clin Psychol 2009;77(3):383.

64. March JS, Silva S, Petrycki S, et al. Fluoxetine, cognitive-behavioral therapy, and their combination for adolescents with depression: treatment for adolescents with depression study (TADS) randomized controlled trial. JAMA 2004;292(7):807–20.

65. Hollon SD, Garber J, Shelton RC. Treatment of depression in adolescents with cognitive behavior therapy and medications: a commentary on the TADS project. Cogn Behav Pract 2005;12(2):149–55.

66. March JS, Silva S, Petrycki S, et al. The treatment for adolescents with depression study (TADS): long-term effectiveness and safety outcomes. Arch Gen Psychiatry 2007;64(10):1132–43.

67. Angold A, Costello EJ, Erkanli A. Comorbidity. J Child Psychol Psychiatry 1999; 40(1):57–87.

68. Rapee RM, Lyneham HJ, Hudson JL, et al. Effect of comorbidity on treatment of anxious children and adolescents: results from a large, combined sample. J Am Acad Child Adolesc Psychiatry 2013;52(1):47–56.

69. Curry J, Rohde P, Simons A, et al. Predictors and moderators of acute outcome in the treatment for adolescents with depression study (TADS). J Am Acad Child Adolesc Psychiatry 2006;45(12):1427–39.

70. Ehrenreich JT, Goldstein CR, Wright LR, et al. Development of a unified protocol for the treatment of emotional disorders in youth. Child Fam Behav Ther 2009; 31(1):20–37.

71. Ehrenreich-May J, Chu BC. Overview of transdiagnostic mechanisms and treatments for youth psychopathology. In: Ehrenreich-May J, Chu BC, editors. Transdiagnostic treatments for children and adolescents: principles and practices. New York: Guilford Press; 2013. p. 3–14.

72. Bilek EL, Ehrenreich-May J. An open trial investigation of a transdiagnostic group treatment for children with anxiety and depressive symptoms. Behav Ther 2012; 43(4):887–97.

73. Chu BC, Crocco ST, Esseling P, et al. Transdiagnostic group behavioral activation and exposure therapy for youth anxiety and depression: initial randomized controlled trial. Behav Res Ther 2016;76:65–75.

74. Kendall PC, Settipani CA, Cummings CM. No need to worry: the promising future of child anxiety research. J Clin Child Adolesc Psychol 2012;41(1):103–15.

75. Weisz JR, McCarty CA, Valeri SM. Effects of psychotherapy for depression in children and adolescents: a meta-analysis. Psychol Bull 2006;132(1):132.

76. Cristea IA, Mogoaşe C, David D, et al. Practitioner review: cognitive bias modification for mental health problems in children and adolescents: a meta-analysis. J Child Psychol Psychiatry 2015;56(7):723–34.

77. MacLeod C, Mathews A. Cognitive bias modification approaches to anxiety. Annu Rev Clin Psychol 2012;8:189–217.

78. Ng MY, Weisz JR. Annual research review: building a science of personalized intervention for youth mental health. J Child Psychol Psychiatry 2016;57(3): 216–36.

79. Chorpita BF, Weisz JR. Modular approach to therapy for children with anxiety, depression, trauma, or conduct problems (MATCH-ADTC). Satellite Beach (FL): PracticeWise LLC; 2009.

80. Weisz JR, Chorpita BF, Palinkas LA, et al. Testing standard and modular designs for psychotherapy treating depression, anxiety, and conduct problems in youth: a randomized effectiveness trial. Arch Gen Psychiatry 2012;69(3):274–82.
81. Ebert DD, Zarski AC, Christensen H, et al. Internet and computer-based cognitive behavioral therapy for anxiety and depression in youth: a meta-analysis of randomized controlled outcome trials. PLoS One 2015;10(3):e0119895.
82. Vigerland S, Lenhard F, Bonnert M, et al. Internet-delivered cognitive behavior therapy for children and adolescents: a systematic review and meta-analysis. Clin Psychol Rev 2016;50:1–10.

Transdiagnostic Therapy

Peter J. Norton, PhD[a],*, Pasquale Roberge, PhD[b]

KEYWORDS

- Transdiagnostic • Comorbidity • Anxiety • Depression
- Cognitive–behavioral therapy

KEY POINTS

- Transdiagnostic cognitive–behavioral therapy (CBT) is designed to be applicable to patients experiencing a range of anxiety and related emotional diagnoses, including those with comorbid emotional disorders.
- Data from clinical trials and metaanalyses support the efficacy of transdiagnostic CBT.
- Transdiagnostic CBT may be more efficacious in treating multiply comorbid presentations.
- Additional comparative outcome trials and studies examining efficacy with obsessive–compulsive disorder and posttraumatic stress disorder are needed.

TRANSDIAGNOSTIC THERAPY

The American Psychological Association's Society of Clinical Psychology (Division 12) maintains a regularly updated database of psychotherapies deemed to meet evidentiary standards to be considered *Research Supported Psychological Therapies*. Within the anxiety and related disorders, cognitive therapy, behavioral therapy, or cognitive–behavioral therapy (CBT) are considered to have strong research support, defined as treatments for which "well-designed studies conducted by independent investigators must converge to support a treatment's efficacy" (https://www.div12.org/psychological-treatments/frequently-asked-questions/; accessed 7 September, 2016). Currently, these include (1) CBT for panic disorder, (2) CBT for social anxiety disorder, (3) CBT for generalized anxiety disorder (GAD), (4) behavior therapy for specific phobias, (5) both cognitive processing therapy and prolonged exposure therapy for posttraumatic stress disorder, and (6) both exposure and response prevention therapy and cognitive therapy for obsessive–compulsive disorder.

Disclosure Statement: The authors have nothing to disclose.
[a] School of Psychological Sciences, Monash University, 18 Innovation Walk, Clayton Campus, Clayton, Victoria 3800 Australia; [b] Department of Family Medicine and Emergency Medicine, Faculty of Medicine and Health Sciences, Université de Sherbrooke, 3001, 12th Avenue North, Sherbrooke, Québec J1H 5N4 Canada
* Corresponding author.
E-mail address: peter.norton@monash.edu

Psychiatr Clin N Am 40 (2017) 675–687
http://dx.doi.org/10.1016/j.psc.2017.08.003
0193-953X/17/© 2017 Elsevier Inc. All rights reserved.

Abbreviations	
CBT	Cognitive–behavioral therapy
DSM	Diagnostic and Statistical Manual of Mental Disorders
GAD	Generalized anxiety disorder

Each of these research-supported therapies contains either cognitive restructuring or exposure, or in most cases, both combined.[1] And yet each intervention is considered distinct, thus requiring the use of and training in at least 6 different protocols to effectively treat the range of anxiety and related disorders.[2] In response, multiple research teams have developed and tested the efficacy of transdiagnostic CBT approaches that incorporate cognitive restructuring and exposure in a diagnosis-independent manner to be broadly efficacious across the anxiety and related disorders.[2–5]

Although variations exist, they all coalesce around the conceptualization that the differences in the fear-eliciting stimuli (eg, public speaking, contamination, traumatic memories) and the typical coping strategies (eg, behavioral withdrawal, rituals, cognitive avoidance) are secondary to the processes underlying the fears. Across diagnoses, anxiety disorders are characterized by similar cognitive processes, such as exaggerated threat-related beliefs regarding the eliciting stimuli, and behavioral processes including conditioned fear response upon presentation of the fear-eliciting stimulus and operant reinforcement of coping behaviors that reduce the fear.[6,7] As such, cognitive strategies such as cognitive restructuring facilitate the reduction of threat-related beliefs, and behavioral techniques such as exposure (incorporating response prevention) serve to reduce the conditioned fear response and accompanying safety behaviors.[8] According to transdiagnostic models of anxiety, transdiagnostic CBT is defined as "[treatments] that apply to the same underlying treatment principles across mental disorders, without tailoring the protocol to specific diagnoses."[9(pp3,4)]

RATIONALE FOR TRANSDIAGNOSTIC COGNITIVE–BEHAVIORAL THERAPY

The case for a transdiagnostic perspective to anxiety disorders[6,10] is founded on (1) arguments regarding the dissemination and accessibility of CBT, (2) the clinical presentation of anxiety and depressive disorders, and (3) the structure of emotional disorders.[11]

Dissemination and Accessibility of Diagnosis-Specific Cognitive–Behavioral Therapy

The increasing complexity of the classification of anxiety disorders has led to the development and refinement of diagnosis-specific CBT treatment protocols that emphasize the distinct clinical characteristics of each disorder. Practitioners are faced with multiple evidence-based psychological treatment protocols for each anxiety disorder that respectively require extensive training and supervision to be delivered with competence and fidelity.[12,13] Unsurprisingly, evidence suggests that these diagnosis-specific treatments are often unavailable or suboptimally delivered in practice.[14]

Transdiagnostic CBT has the potential to improve the quality of care for patients with anxiety disorders through more efficient dissemination of CBT in clinical practice. Among the advantages associated with transdiagnostic CBT, limited resources are required for training and supervision, because the approach moves away from the multiple diagnosis-specific treatment protocols toward overarching transdiagnostic CBT manualized protocols well-suited to the reality of clinical settings.[10,14,15] Furthermore, advances in the delivery of transdiagnostic CBT have focused on alternatives to resource-intensive conventional psychotherapy to support optimal allocation of highly qualified mental health specialists in the context of limited resources and expertise, with treatment modalities such as group[2] or Internet-delivered transdiagnostic CBT.[16] These treatment modalities are also increasingly amenable to the delivery in community mental health settings, where patients' clinical profiles are heterogeneous.[10,14,15]

Comorbidity, Not Otherwise Specified, and Complex Presentations

Based on clinical and epidemiologic surveys, approximately half of patients with a principal diagnosis of anxiety disorder also meet criteria for at least one additional co-morbid anxiety or depressive disorder, which means that complex clinical profiles are seen in practice more often than single diagnosis presentations.[17,18] Comorbidity has consequences on both the conceptualization of emotional disorders and treatment decisions, such as treating one disorder, combining or delivering sequentially diagnosis-specific treatments, or adopting a concurrent transdiagnostic CBT approach. A transdiagnostic CBT seems to be particularly promising for managing co-morbidity.[19] In primary care, where psychiatric comorbidity is the norm, the differential diagnosis of anxiety disorders is often uncertain and the anxiety disorder not otherwise specified (*Diagnostic and Statistical Manual of Mental Disorders* [DSM]-IV) or unspecified/other–specified anxiety disorder (DSM-5) diagnoses are common.[20,21] Currently, no psychological therapies are considered research supported for the treatment of "not otherwise specified" or other catchall diagnostic categories.

Match with Structural Models of Anxiety

Although variations exist, transdiagnostic models of anxiety[7,22] and emotional disorders more broadly[6] hold that the similarities across the different diagnoses outweigh the differences. Considerable work across a number of domains, including genetics, neurobiology, learning theory, cognitive science, and developmental psychology, highlight substantial key commonalities across diagnoses with much less evidence suggesting diagnosis-specific factors. In summarizing the genetic literature, Smoller and colleagues[23] conclude that "evidence from a range of studies suggests that genetic influences transcend the boundaries of the DSM categories."[(p121)] This is supported by twin epidemiologic studies,[24] and preliminary suggestions from candidate gene association and genome-wide association studies,[23,25] which indicate that genetic susceptibility to anxiety and other negative emotional disorders is not diagnosis specific, and may represent a single (or potentially dual[24]) transdiagnostic influence toward the development of any anxiety or depressive disorder.

Similarly, from a neurologic perspective the evidence is generally supportive of a transdiagnostic conceptualization. Across studies, although various structures and pathways have been implicated separately for different anxiety disorder diagnoses,[26] the central role of the amygdalocortical circuitry is maintained.[27] However, cross-diagnosis comparisons of the role of either the amygdala or other structures, have been few making it difficult to ascertain the extent to which neurologic data support either a transdiagnostic framework or a DSM-like (or other) distinction between diagnoses. In one such cross-diagnosis comparison, using a sample of participants with GAD, panic disorder, social anxiety disorder, and healthy controls, Fonzo and colleagues[28] used functional MRI during a facial emotion matching task. Results showed identical activation (compared with healthy controls) in the amygdala after presentation of fearful faces. Increased activity in the posterior insula was observed among only participants with panic disorder, and left posterior temporal regions showed greater activation among participants with panic disorder and social anxiety disorder, but not GAD, suggesting the possibility of both transdiagnostic and diagnosis-specific patterns of neurologic involvement. Even so, according to Britton and Rauch,[27] "given the similarities in some symptoms across anxiety disorders, a common underlying neural correlate is expected to subserve the shared symptom profile of anxiety."[(p97)]

From the perspective of developmental psychology, the majority of the literature examining developmental risks and pathways to developing an anxiety disorder suggest no factors that differentially mediate the development of one anxiety disorder over another. Indeed, the most thoroughly studied developmental factors underlying anxiety disorders, including temperamental variables such as behavioral inhibition and neuroticism, parenting styles including controlling/overprotectiveness, parental characteristics such as lack of emotional warmth, childhood adversity, and the quality of the parent–child attachment, have little to no differential association with specific childhood or adult anxiety disorder diagnoses.[29]

When examining the behavioral and cognitive variables associated with anxiety disorders, few differences in acquisition or maintenance properties have been noted. For example, considerable evidence links attentional biases for threat-related information with each anxiety diagnosis, but little evidence suggests that the strength or nature of the threat bias differs across fears.[30,31] Similarly, behavioral fear acquisition and maintenance mechanisms do not differ across fears or diagnoses. There is some evidence that certain "prepared" fears—fears of stimuli that have an evolutionary threat relevance—may more easily acquired or maintained,[32] although this conclusion is equivocal.[33] Even so, the distinction between prepared and unprepared stimuli is not inherent in DSM anxiety disorder diagnostic classifications.

Finally, treatment data tend to offer support for a transdiagnostic formulation of anxiety disorders, because the evidence suggests comparable response to highly similar treatments across diagnoses. CBT approaches incorporating cognitive restructuring and exposure, for example, have been shown in 2 separate metaanalyses to result in comparable effect sizes across panic disorder, social anxiety disorder, obsessive–compulsive disorder, posttraumatic stress disorder, and GAD.[1,34] Serotonergic medications, particularly paroxetine and sertraline, have US Food and Drug Administration indications at similar or identical doses across the major anxiety disorder diagnoses (sertraline does not carry current US Food and Drug Administration indication for GAD, and neither sertraline nor paroxetine is indicated for specific phobias).[35,36]

Together, evidence supporting a shared etiology and high rates of current and lifetime comorbidity within anxiety disorders and with mood disorders are consistent with a latent structure, a common higher order pathology. A paradigm shift toward a transdiagnostic, or unified, conceptualization of anxiety disorders seems appropriate because it is supported by empirical findings pointing toward a common pathology of anxiety disorders, and is a promising gateway to improve access to CBT in community settings.

PREPARATION FOR TRANSDIAGNOSTIC COGNITIVE–BEHAVIORAL THERAPY: ASSESSMENT AND CASE FORMULATION

Although the knowledge base on the transdiagnostic case conceptualization and treatment of emotional disorders is growing rapidly, the development of transdiagnostic measures that reflect a common pathology framework is not evolving at the same pace.[37] The emphasis on categorical diagnostic classification systems (ie, DSM-5, *International Classification of Diseases*-10) has led to the development of clinician-rated structured interviews, including the commonly used Structured Clinical Interview for DSM-5[38] and Anxiety Disorders Interview Schedule for DSM-5,[39] as well as numerous self-report questionnaires that provide valuable clinical information for research and practice. However, assessment tools based on discrete diagnostic entities present limitations for use in a transdiagnostic model because they do not inform us on the underlying core processes that may be associated with the development and maintenance of emotional disorders.[37,40] Furthermore, as Smith and colleagues[37] emphasize, transdiagnostic assessment could benefit from overall severity and interference scores to account for the additive effects of comorbid anxiety and related disorders. With the publication of the Anxiety Disorders Interview Schedule for DSM-5[39] a qualitative (0–8) "overall distress/impairment" scale has been implemented to augment the severity ratings of each diagnosis, although this clinician rating does not seem to be specific to anxiety diagnoses.

Cognitive–behavioral case formulation is a valuable framework to guide clinical assessment and treatment planning within a transdiagnostic model. Derived in part from behavioral assessment, case formulation-driven CBT is tailored to each patient and aims at developing hypothesis about underlying mechanisms associated with the development and maintenance of mental health problems and maladaptive functioning.[41] The transdiagnostic case formulation, leading to treatment planning and outcome assessment, relies on clinical interviews and observations, as well as self-report assessment tools.[41,42] There are several self-reported assessment tools that can be beneficial to assess global anxiety and depression, specific symptoms, construct-based psychological mechanisms, and quality of life and functional impairment.[37,43]

Common self-reported measures of global anxiety severity include the Beck Anxiety Inventory,[44] the State-Trait Anxiety Inventory,[45] and the Depression, Anxiety, and Stress Scales.[46] Although these tools are brief, reliable, and allow for comparison across transdiagnostic and diagnosis-specific studies, they are often biased toward specific anxiety features. To address the lack of assessment tools for multiple anxiety disorders, Norman and colleagues[47] developed and validated the Overall Anxiety Severity and Impairment Scale, a 5-item measure assessing global anxiety disorder severity over a past-week duration.[47–49] More recently, Norton and Robinson[43] developed the Anxiety Disorder Diagnostic Questionnaire to assess fear, anxiety/worry, perceived interference, and distress and anxiety symptoms across diagnosis. The monthly and weekly Anxiety Disorder Diagnostic Questionnaire shows good psychometric properties.[43,50]

IMPLEMENTING TRANSDIAGNOSTIC COGNITIVE–BEHAVIORAL THERAPY

At their core, most transdiagnostic CBT protocols incorporate psychoeducation and some degree of cognitive restructuring and exposure therapy, although variations in the intensity and target of each approach exist across transdiagnostic CBT protocols. A general transdiagnostic CBT framework is presented here, followed by specific variations within the most well-studied treatment protocols.

Psychoeducation provides factual information regarding the nature and causes of anxiety disorders, as well as an explanation of how the intervention components are designed to target different maintaining aspects of the anxiety. Common psychoeducational elements include, but are certainly not limited to, (1) an explanation of genetic, developmental, and experiential vulnerability factors underlying anxiety disorders, (2) a discussion of the interplay between cognitions physiologic responses, and safety motivations, and their adaptive functions, (3) self-monitoring of anxiety or specific responses, and (4) a discussion of the treatment rationale from a behavioral, cognitive, or combined cognitive–behavioral framework.

Cognitive restructuring refers to a collection of methods and techniques designed to assist clients in identifying biased or inaccurate perceptions of fear or anxiety-provoking stimuli, based on cognitive models that propose that anxiety disorder (eg, fear of public speaking) exists as a function of biased or distorted beliefs about the situation or its consequences (eg, "I will humiliate myself") rather than actual properties of the situation or stimulus itself (eg, the audience). Cognitive restructuring approaches involve the identification of anxious appraisals, evaluating biases or distortions such as catastrophizing or overestimation of probabilities, and generating more realistic appraisals of the anxiety-provoking situation or stimulus.

Exposure therapy, borne out of behavioral models of fear acquisition, maintenance, and extinction, typically involve the gradual confrontation of the fear-provoking situations or stimuli—from easier to more difficult—to promote habituation to the situations or stimuli over multiple exposure sessions. As a simple example, an exposure plan for an individual with a fear of spiders might begin with pictures of spiders, followed by a rubber spider, a live spider in a sealed terrarium, a live spider in an open-topped terrarium and, finally, a live spider held in the patient's palm. Although frequently only made explicit in exposure therapy for obsessive–compulsive disorder, response prevention—the client's voluntary withholding of safety behaviors—is seen as essential for safety learning and cognitive reevaluation of threat during exposures.

Many diagnosis-specific CBT protocols stipulate specific forms of exposure therapy, including interoceptive exposure to feared bodily sensations (eg, CBT for panic disorder), in vivo exposures to external stimuli or situations (eg, CBT for specific phobias), or imaginal exposure to worries (eg, CBT for GAD), intrusive thoughts (eg, CBT for obsessive–compulsive disorder), or traumatic memories (eg, CBT for posttraumatic stress disorder). In transdiagnostic CBT protocols, however, the emphasis is not on the prescription of specific formats of exposure. but rather on identifying and flexibly applying exposure techniques that achieve the function of provoking client anxiety in a graduated fashion. As such, exposure plans can be formulated based on the specific feared situations or stimuli of each particular client rather than prototypical clients with a specific diagnosis. Further, a transdiagnostic approach to exposure therapy may be more parsimonious for clients with comorbid anxiety diagnoses.

In the Transdiagnostic Group CBT[2] protocol, the treatment elements of psychoeducation, cognitive restructuring, and exposure therapy are incorporated largely as described. Psychoeducation is delivered in the first session, and cognitive restructuring is introduced and practices in sessions 2 and 3. Sessions 4 through 9 involve graduated exposure therapy. Specific to the Norton protocol,[2] sessions 10 and 11 shift to cognitive restructuring techniques applied to broader schema-level beliefs, and the final session addresses relapse prevention and termination issues.

The Barlow and colleagues[3] Unified Protocol likewise contains cognitive and exposure treatment elements, although the emphasis of exposure and response prevention is on reducing emotional avoidance and emotion-driven behaviors through exposure-like activities. Rather than specific session-by-session content, the Barlow and colleagues[3] protocol is organized into 8 ordered modules that can be applied flexibly across multiple sessions, depending on client treatment progress. The primary modules include emotional awareness, appraisal flexibility, prevention of avoidance, and exposure, and may be augmented by modules emphasizing motivational enhancement, understanding emotions, tolerating physical sensations, and relapse prevention.

Other promising transdiagnostic CBT protocols have been developed, albeit with less developed research evidence support. Schmidt and colleagues,[5] for example, developed a brief transdiagnostic CBT protocol focusing predominantly on exposure and response prevention, and without any cognitive restructuring component. Originally evaluated in a 10-session format[5] but shortened to 5 sessions in a later study,[51] their protocol emphasizes reduction and elimination of safety behaviors, such as avoidance or compulsions, and engagement in antiphobic behaviors through situational, interoceptive, and cognitive exposure activities. Nathan and associates[52] developed a 10-session transdiagnostic group CBT designed for individuals with anxiety and depression. The protocol predominantly uses cognitive restructuring, exposure, and behavioral activation, as well as incorporation of relaxation and calming techniques. Other investigators have developed additional transdiagnostic CBT programs for anxiety disorders,[53–55] although efficacy data supporting these protocols remain limited. Although outside of the scope of this paper, other researchers[16] have developed and evaluated Internet-based approaches to transdiagnostic CBT with encouraging data from several trials.[56]

EMPIRICAL OUTCOMES DATA ON TRANSDIAGNOSTIC COGNITIVE–BEHAVIORAL THERAPY

Given the general paucity of follow-up outcome studies for transdiagnostic CBT, the available published data on the efficacy of transdiagnostic CBT for anxiety disorders will be broken down into, first, short-term or immediate posttreatment outcomes, followed by the limited available longer term outcomes.

Short-term Outcomes

Across multiple studies conducted by independent research teams, immediate posttreatment outcomes for transdiagnostic CBT are highly encouraging. Multiple open trials have reported significant posttreatment reductions in self-reported anxiety or clinician-rated anxiety disorder severity.[4,57–60] Further, randomized clinical trials comparing against no treatment waitlist controls have found that such improvement is not attributable to spontaneous remission or other nontherapy factors.[5,61–65] These data are buttressed by several metaanalyses of transdiagnostic CBT converging on the conclusion that transdiagnostic CBT is associated with large reductions in anxiety disorder symptoms and severity.[10,66–69] Beyond symptom and diagnostic severity, indices of quality of life also show improvement after transdiagnostic CBT.[70,71]

Most important, one randomized clinical trial comparing transdiagnostic CBT with other established psychotherapy approaches—including applied relaxation and diagnosis-specific CBT—have reported statistical equivalence[64,65] between the treatments at posttreatment. Finally, a recent metaanalysis indicated small but statistically significantly larger ($P = .008$) uncontrolled pretreatment to posttreatment anxiety reduction effect sizes in clinical trials of transdiagnostic CBT (Hedges' $g = 1.06$) in comparison with clinical trials of diagnosis-specific CBT (Hedges' $g = 0.95$).[68]

Long-term Outcomes

Despite the encouraging posttreatment efficacy data, only 2 long-term follow-up studies have been conducted. Dwyer and colleagues[57] reported no significant change on measures of clinical outcomes from posttreatment to 12-month follow-up in their open trial of 2 transdiagnostic CBT protocols for anxiety and depression, respectively. Unfortunately, data were not separated for those enrolled in the transdiagnostic CBT for anxiety and transdiagnostic CBT for depression conditions, so it is unclear the extent to which the maintenance of gains was common or unique to 1 protocol. Similarly, using a small subsample (n = 15) of patients from several studies, Bullis and colleagues[72] reported that treatment gains were maintained at 6-month and at longer term (12- to 24-month) follow-up.

Effects on Comorbid Diagnoses

Given the presumed benefits of transdiagnostic CBT on comorbid presentations, several studies have examined rates of remission of nonprincipal comorbid diagnoses after transdiagnostic CBT. Norton and colleagues[19] conducted a secondary analysis of participant data from 3 trials and reported that 67% of participants with multiple diagnoses showed remission of all comorbid DSM-IV axis I diagnoses to subclinical levels. These data were benchmarked against 7 trials of diagnosis-specific CBT for specific anxiety disorders wherein an average comorbid diagnosis remission rate of 41.36%. Similarly, although Ellard and colleagues[58] did not compute remission rates, they reported that 64% of participants achieved high end-state functioning status for comorbid diagnoses after transdiagnostic CBT. When examining comorbid DSM-IV diagnoses of major depressive disorder, dysthymic disorder, or depressive disorder not otherwise specified, Talkovsky and colleagues[73] reported an immediate posttreatment rate of depressive diagnosis remission to subclinical levels of 71.4%.

Modified transdiagnostic CBT interventions have been developed in an effort to address additional common comorbidities, including comorbid anxiety and chronic headache in adolescents,[74] mood, anxiety, and substance use disorders,[75] and bipolar disorder with comorbid anxiety.[76] However, data for each are still preliminary and require replication. Even so, transdiagnostic CBT seems to be advantageous for integrated interventional approaches, as diagnosis-specific approaches would become burdensome to meet the necessary permutations with each DSM-5 anxiety disorder.

SUMMARY AND FUTURE DIRECTIONS

As noted elsewhere,[77] transdiagnostic CBT for anxiety and related disorder has undergone considerable growth over the past 2 decades since the initial theoretic models[6] and trials were published.[55,78] For 2016, the Scopus database (accessed 14 February, 2017) returns 83 documents containing the search terms "(Transdiagnostic) AND (Anxiety) AND ((Therapy) or (Intervention))", suggesting widespread investigation into these interventions. Transdiagnostic CBT approaches for multiple and comorbid anxiety disorder diagnoses has shown efficacy across multiple open trials,[4,57–60] randomized, controlled trials by comparison with waitlist controls,[5,61–63] and metaanalyses,[10,66–69] statistically equivalent—and perhaps superior—outcomes in comparison to existing research-supporting diagnosis-specific CBT approaches,[65,68] and superior efficacy to diagnosis-specific CBT in treating comorbid anxiety diagnoses.[19,58]

Although encouraging, several key areas of investigation are required. First, and perhaps most important, long-term follow-up data are urgently required; only 2 studies have reported outcomes beyond the immediate posttreatment period.[57,72] Second, additional demonstrations of the comparative efficacy of transdiagnostic CBT and diagnosis-specific CBT are required, with only 1 small randomized, controlled trial[65] and 1 metaanalytic comparison[68] published thus far. One large trial comparing transdiagnostic CBT has been completed and data are forthcoming (Barlow DH, Farchione TJ, Bullis JR et al, A randomized equivalence evaluation of the Unified Protocol for Transdiagnostic Treatment of Emotional Disorders compared with diagnosis-specific CBT for anxiety disorders. Submitted for publication.). Finally, the majority of the efficacy data have come from samples consisting primarily of panic disorder, social anxiety disorder, and GAD. It is, therefore, imperative that additional trials examining the efficacy of transdiagnostic CBT approaches with posttraumatic stress disorder and obsessive–compulsive disorder. Limitations aside, as noted by Meidlinger and Hope[11] in a recent review of the transdiagnostic CBT literature, "transdiagnostic treatments offer a number of appealing advantages to the mental health field such as better matching research-driven models of mental health problems, health care system advantages such as improved ease of dissemination, and basic clinical advantages such as improvements in the ability to address comorbidity."[(p7)]

REFERENCES

1. Norton PJ, Price EP. A meta-analytic review of cognitive-behavioral treatment outcome across the anxiety disorders. J Nerv Ment Dis 2007;195:521–31.

2. Norton PJ. Group cognitive-behavioral therapy of anxiety: a transdiagnostic treatment manual. New York: Guilford; 2012.

3. Barlow DH, Farchione TJ, Fairholme CP, et al. Unified protocol for transdiagnostic treatment of emotional disorders: therapist guide. New York: Oxford University Press; 2011.

4. Gros DF. Development and initial evaluation of transdiagnostic behavior therapy (TBT) for veterans with affective disorders. Psychiatry Res 2013;220:275–82.

5. Schmidt NB, Buckner JD, Pusser A, et al. Randomized controlled trial of false safety behavior elimination therapy: a unified cognitive behavioral treatment for anxiety psychopathology. Behav Ther 2012;43:518–32.

6. Barlow DH, Allen LB, Choate ML. Toward a unified treatment for emotional disorders. Behav Ther 2004;35:205–30.

7. Norton PJ. Toward a clinically-oriented model of anxiety disorders. Cogn Behav Ther 2006;35:88–105.

8. Norton PJ, Paulus DJ. Towards a unified treatment for emotional disorders: update on the science and practice. Behav Ther 2016;47:854–68.

9. McEvoy PM, Nathan P, Norton PJ. Efficacy of transdiagnostic treatments: a review of published outcome studies and future research directions. J Cogn Psychother 2009;23:20–33.

10. Norton PJ, Philipp LM. Transdiagnostic approaches to the treatment of anxiety disorders: a quantitative review. Psychotherapy (Chic) 2008;45:214–26.

11. Meidlinger PC, Hope DA. The new transdiagnostic cognitive behavioral treatments: commentary for clinicians and clinical researchers. J Anxiety Disord 2017;46:101–9.

12. Farchione TJ, Bullis JR. Addressing the global burden of mental illness: why transdiagnostic and common elements approaches to evidence-based practice might be our best bet. Cogn Behav Pract 2014;21:124–6.

13. Gunter RW, Whittal ML. Dissemination of cognitive-behavioral treatments for anxiety disorders: overcoming barriers and improving patient access. Clin Psychol Rev 2010;30:194–202.

14. Shafran R, Clark DM, Fairburn CG, et al. Mind the gap: improving the dissemination of CBT. Behav Res Ther 2009;47:902–9.

15. Clark DA. Cognitive behavioral therapy for anxiety and depression: possibilities and limitations of a transdiagnostic perspective. Cogn Behav Ther 2009;38:29–34.

16. Titov N, Andrews G, Johnston L, et al. Transdiagnostic internet treatment for anxiety disorders: a randomized controlled trial. Behav Res Ther 2010;48:890–9.

17. Lamers F, van Oppen P, Comijs HC, et al. Comorbidity patterns of anxiety and depressive disorders in a large cohort study: the Netherlands Study of Depression and Anxiety (NESDA). J Clin Psychiatry 2011;72:341–8.
18. Kessler RC, Chiu WT, Demler O, et al. Prevalence, severity, and comorbidity of twelve-month DSM-IV disorders in the national comorbidity survey replication (NCS- R). Arch Gen Psychiatry 2005;62:617–27.
19. Norton PJ, Barrera TL, Mathew AR, et al. Effect of transdiagnostic CBT for anxiety on comorbid diagnoses. Depress Anxiety 2013;30:168–73.
20. Boulenger JP, Fournier M, Rosales D, et al. Mixed anxiety and depression: from theory to practice. J Clin Psychiatry 1997;58(Suppl. 8):27–34.
21. Kroenke K, Spitzer RL, Williams JB, et al. Anxiety disorders in primary care: prevalence, impairment, comorbidity, and detection. Ann Intern Med 2007;146: 317–25.
22. Norton PJ, Paulus DJ. Transdiagnostic models of anxiety disorder: theoretical and empirical underpinnings. Clin Psychol Rev 2017;56:122–37.
23. Smoller JW, Gardner-Schuster E, Covino J. The genetic basis of panic and phobic anxiety disorders. Am J Med Genet C Semin Med Genet 2008;148C: 140–7.
24. Hettema JM, Prescott CA, Myers JM, et al. The structure of genetic and environmental risk factors for anxiety disorders in men and women. Arch Gen Psychiatry 2005;62:182–9.
25. Hettema JM. What is the genetic relationship between anxiety and depression? Am J Med Genet C Semin Med Genet 2008;148C:140–7.
26. Gray JA, McNaughton N. The neuropsychology of anxiety: an enquiry into the function of the septo-hippocampal system. 2nd edition. New York: Oxford University Press; 2000.
27. Britton JC, Rauch SL. Neuroanatomy and neuroimaging of anxiety disorders. In: Antony MM, Stein MB, editors. Oxford handbook of anxiety and related disorders. New York: Oxford University Press; 2009. p. 97–110.
28. Fonzo GA, Ramsawh HJ, Flagan TM, et al. Common and disorder-specific neural responses to emotional faces in generalised anxiety, social anxiety and panic disorders. Br J Psychiatry 2015;206:206–15.
29. Beesdo K, Knappe S, Pine DS. Anxiety and anxiety disorders in children and adolescents: developmental issues and implications for DSM-V. Psychiatr Clin North Am 2009;32:483–524.
30. Cisler JM, Koster EH. Mechanisms of attentional biases towards threat in anxiety disorders: an integrative review. Clin Psychol Rev 2010;30:203–16.
31. McNally RJ, Reese HE. Information processing approaches to understanding anxiety disorders. In: Antony MM, Stein MB, editors. Oxford handbook of anxiety and related disorders. New York: Oxford University Press; 2009. p. 136–52.
32. Seligman MEP. Phobias and preparedness. Behav Ther 1971;2:307–20.
33. McNally RJ. The legacy of Seligman's "Phobias and Preparedness" (1971). Behav Ther 2016;47:585–94.
34. Hofmann SG, Smits JAJ. Cognitive-behavioral therapy for adult anxiety disorders: a meta-analysis of randomized placebo-controlled trials. J Clin Psychiatry 2008; 69:621–32.
35. Melton ST, Kirkwood CK. Anxiety disorders I: generalized anxiety, panic, and social anxiety disorders. In: DiPiro JT, Talbert RL, Yee GC, et al, editors. Pharmacotherapy: a pathophysiologic approach. 9th edition. New York: McGraw Hill; 2014.

36. Kirkwood CK, Melton ST, Wells BG. Anxiety disorders II: posttraumatic stress disorder and obsessive-compulsive disorder. In: DiPiro JT, Talbert RL, Yee GC, et al, editors. Pharmacotherapy: a pathophysiologic approach. 9th edition. McGraw Hill: New York; 2014.

37. Smith AH, Ratcliff C, Norton PJ. Transdiagnostic cognitive assessment and case formulation for anxiety: a new approach. In: Clark DA, Brown GP, editors. Assessment in cognitive therapy. New York: Guilford; 2014. p. 197–220.

38. First MB, Williams JBW, Karg RS, et al. Structured clinical interview for DSM-5—research version(SCID-5 for DSM-5, research version; SCID-5-RV). Arlington (VA): American Psychiatric Association; 2015.

39. Brown TA, Barlow DH. Anxiety and related disorders interview schedule for DSM-5 (ADIS-5) - adult and lifetime version: clinician manual. New York: Oxford University Press; 2014.

40. Mansell W, Harvey A, Watkins E, et al. Conceptual foundations of the transdiagnostic approach to CBT. J Cogn Psychother 2009;23:6–19.

41. Persons JB. The case formulation approach to cognitive-behavior therapy. New York: Guilford Press; 2008.

42. Frank RI, Davidson J. The transdiagnostic roadmap to case formulation and treatment planning: practical guidance for clinical decision making. Oakland (CA): New Harbinger Publications; 2014.

43. Norton PJ, Robinson CM. Development and evaluation of the anxiety disorder diagnostic questionnaire. Cogn Behav Ther 2010;39:137–49.

44. Beck AT, Epstein N, Brown G, et al. An inventory for measuring clinical anxiety: psychometric properties. J Consult Clin Psychol 1988;56:893–7.

45. Spielberger CD, Gorsuch RL, Luschene RE, et al. State-trait anxiety inventory for adults. Palo Alto (CA): Mind Garden; 1983.

46. Lovibond SH, Lovibond PF. Manual for the depression, anxiety and stress scales. 2nd edition. Sydney (Australia): Psychology Foundation; 1995.

47. Norman SB, Cissell SH, Means-Christensen AJ, et al. Development and validation of an overall anxiety severity and impairment scale (OASIS). Depress Anxiety 2006;23:245–9.

48. Campbell-Sills L, Norman SB, Craske MG, et al. Validation of a brief measure of anxiety-related severity and impairment: the overall anxiety severity and impairment scale (OASIS). J Affect Disord 2009;112:92–101.

49. Bragdon LB, Diefenbach GJ, Hannan S, et al. Psychometric properties of the overall anxiety severity and impairment scale (OASIS) among psychiatric outpatients. J Affect Disord 2016;201:112–5.

50. Smith AH, Paulus DJ, Norton PJ. Transdiagnostic assessment of anxiety symptoms using the anxiety disorder diagnostic questionnaire - weekly version. Anxiety Stress Coping 2017;30:96–106.

51. Riccardi CJ, Korte KJ, Schmidt NB. False safety behavior elimination therapy: a randomized study of a brief individual transdiagnostic treatment for anxiety disorders. J Anxiety Disord 2017;46:35–45.

52. Nathan PR, Rees CS, Smith LM. Mood management course: a group cognitive behavioural programme for anxiety disorders and depression. Perth (Australia): Rioby; 2001. Available at: http://www.cci.health.wa.gov.au/index.html.

53. Larkin KT, Waller S, Combs-Lane A. Anxiety management group therapy for multiple anxiety disorder diagnoses. In P. J. Norton (Chair), Integrative Treatment Approaches Across Anxiety and Related Disorders. Symposium presented at the annual meeting of the Anxiety Disorders Association of America. Toronto, ON, March 29, 2003.

54. Garcia MS. Effectiveness of cognitive-behavioural group therapy in patients with anxiety disorders. Psychol Spain 2004;8:89–97.
55. Erickson DH. Group cognitive behavioural therapy for heterogeneous anxiety disorders. Cogn Behav Ther 2003;32:179–86.
56. Newby JM, Mewton L, Andrews G. Transdiagnostic versus disorder-specific internet-delivered cognitive behaviour therapy for anxiety and depression in primary care. J Anxiety Disord 2017;46:25–34.
57. Dwyer L, Olsen S, Oei TPS. Cognitive behavior group therapy for heterogeneous anxiety and depressive disorder in a psychiatric hospital outpatient clinic. J Cogn Psychother 2013;27:138–54.
58. Ellard KK, Fairholme CP, Boisseau CL, et al. Unified protocol for the transdiagnostic treatment of emotional disorders: protocol development and initial outcome data. Cogn Behav Pract 2010;17:88–101.
59. McEvoy PM, Nathan P. Effectiveness of cognitive behavior therapy for diagnostically heterogeneous groups: a benchmarking study. J Consult Clin Psychol 2007; 75:344–50, 66.
60. Oei TPS, Boschen MJ. Clinical effectiveness of a cognitive behavioral group treatment program for anxiety disorders: a benchmarking study. J Anxiety Disord 2009;23:950–7.
61. Erickson DH, Janeck AS, Tallman K. A cognitive-behavioral group for patients with various anxiety disorders. Psychiatr Serv 2007;58:1205–11.
62. Farchione TJ, Fairholme CP, Ellard KK, et al. Unified protocol for transdiagnostic treatment of emotional disorders: a randomized controlled trial. Behav Ther 2012; 43:666–78.
63. Norton PJ, Hope DA. Preliminary evaluation of a broad-spectrum cognitive-behavioral group therapy for anxiety. J Behav Ther Exp Psychiatry 2005;36: 79–97.
64. Norton PJ. A randomized clinical trial of transdiagnostic CBT for anxiety disorder by comparison to relaxation training. Behav Ther 2012;43:506–17.
65. Norton PJ, Barrera TL. Transdiagnostic versus diagnosis-specific CBT for anxiety disorders: a preliminary randomized controlled trial. Depress Anxiety 2012;29: 874–82.
66. Andersen P, Toner P, Bland M, et al. Effectiveness of transdiagnostic cognitive behavior therapy for anxiety and depression in adults: a systematic review and meta-analysis. Behav Cogn Psychother 2016;44:673–90.
67. Newby JM, McKinnon A, Kuyken W, et al. Systematic review and meta-analysis of transdiagnostic psychological treatments for anxiety and depressive disorders in adulthood. Clin Psychol Rev 2015;40:91–110.
68. Pearl S, Norton PJ. Transdiagnostic versus diagnosis specific cognitive behavioural therapies for anxiety: a meta-analysis. J Anxiety Disord 2017;46:11–24.
69. Reinholt N, Krogh J. Efficacy of transdiagnostic cognitive behaviour therapy for anxiety disorders: a systematic review and meta-analysis of published outcome studies. Cogn Behav Ther 2014;43:1–14.
70. Talkovsky AM, Paulus DJ, Kuang F, et al. Quality of life outcomes following transdiagnostic group cognitive-behavioral therapy for anxiety. Int J Cogn Ther 2017; 9:1–22.
71. Gallagher MW, Sauer-Zavala SE, Boswell JF, et al. The impact of the unified protocol for emotional disorders on quality of life. Int J Cogn Ther 2013;6:57–72.
72. Bullis JR, Fortune MR, Farchione TJ, et al. A preliminary investigation of the long-term outcome of the unified protocol for transdiagnostic treatment of emotional disorders. Compr Psychiatry 2014;55:1920–7.

73. Talkovsky AM, Green KL, Osegueda AJ, et al. Transactional effects of depression in transdiagnostic group cognitive behavioral therapy for anxiety. J Anxiety Disord 2017;46:56–64.
74. Sharma P, Mehta M, Sagar R. Efficacy of transdiagnostic cognitive-behavioral group therapy for anxiety disorders and headache in adolescents. J Anxiety Disord 2017;46:78–84.
75. Milosevic I, Chudzic SM, Boyd S, et al. Evaluation of an integrated group cognitive-behavioral treatment for comorbid mood, anxiety, and substance use disorders: a pilot study. J Anxiety Disord 2017;46:85–100.
76. Ellard KK, Deckersbach T, Sylvia LG, et al. Transdiagnostic treatment of bipolar disorder and comorbid anxiety with the unified protocol: a clinical replication series. Behav Modif 2012;36:482–508.
77. Norton PJ. Transdiagnostic approaches to the understanding and treatment of anxiety and related disorders. J Anxiety Disord 2017;46:1–3.
78. Norton PJ, Hayes SA, Hope DA. Effects of a transdiagnostic group treatment for anxiety on secondary depressive disorders. Depress Anxiety 2004;20:198–202.

Internet-Assisted Cognitive Behavioral Therapy

Gerhard Andersson, PhD, Dr Med Sci[a,b],*, Per Carlbring, PhD[c]

KEYWORDS

- Internet-delivered cognitive–behavioral therapy • Anxiety • Mood disorder
- Information technology

KEY POINTS

- The Internet is used by a large number of people and also in health care.
- Cognitive–behavioral therapy (CBT) has been adapted and transferred for Internet delivery.
- A large number of psychiatric conditions can be treated using clinician-assisted Internet treatment.
- An increasing number of studies suggest that guided Internet-based CBT can be as effective as face-to-face CBT.

BACKGROUND

The Internet, including modern information technology, has had a dramatic impact on many areas of life, including health care and psychological treatment. In particular, cognitive–behavioral therapy (CBT) has been found to be a form of psychological treatment that has been possible to transfer to other modes of delivery than regular face-to-face and group formats.[1] The Internet is not only useful for providing CBT, but has a significant role in providing information about CBT and conditions that are treated using CBT.[2] In addition, modern information technology also has a major role in assessment procedures, such as online administration of self-report measures.[3] In this article, we focus mainly on Internet-supported treatments, although another emerging format is to use video conferencing systems[4] and conduct real-time face-to-face CBT, CBT training,[5] or supervision.[6]

Disclosure Statement: The authors have no conflict of interest.
[a] Department of Behavioural Sciences and Learning, Linköping University, Campus Valla, SE-581 83, Linköping SE-581 83, Sweden; [b] Department of Clinical Neuroscience, Karolinska Institute, Stockholm, Sweden; [c] Department of Psychology, Stockholm University, Stockholm SE-106 91, Sweden
* Corresponding author. Department of Behavioural Sciences and Learning, Linköping University, Campus valla, SE-581 83, Linköping SE-581 83, Sweden.
E-mail address: gerhard.andersson@liu.se

Psychiatr Clin N Am 40 (2017) 689–700
http://dx.doi.org/10.1016/j.psc.2017.08.004
0193-953X/17/© 2017 Elsevier Inc. All rights reserved.

psych.theclinics.com

Abbreviations	
CBT	cognitive–behavioral therapy
ICBT	Internet-assisted CBT

The present article has 3 aims. First, we provide a brief description of Internet-assisted CBT (ICBT), and then we review evidence for mood and anxiety disorders. We briefly discuss moderators and mediators of outcome, and end with a discussion about future directions. Given several previous systematic reviews and meta-analyses we only provide examples of programs tested in randomized, controlled trials.

A DIFFERENT WAY TO DO COGNITIVE–BEHAVIORAL THERAPY

The history of ICBT is relatively short and scattered, given the inconsistent terminology and confusion regarding the role of technology versus the role of the supporting clinician.[7] Computers were used early in CBT,[8] but the evidence base grew slowly and use of CD-ROM and other offline formats were more or less abandoned (or at least less popular) when similar programs became available on the Internet. Another background is bibliotherapy and a large number of studies showing that CBT can be described in self-help books for use either supported or unsupported by clinicians.[9] Self-help books are still commonly sold and used, frequently as adjuncts to face-to-face CBT.[10] The first studies on ICBT were published in the late 1990s. One form of ICBT relies heavily on self-help texts and can be referred to as "net bibliotherapy,"[11] even if that term adds even more confusion as the amount of interactive computerized features have varied for as long as ICBT has been around. Herein we describe how ICBT can be delivered and also highlight differences in approaches when motivated. The first necessary component is the treatment platform. Even if there have been numerous published trials on ICBT, there are few descriptions of the platforms behind.[12,13] Briefly, the functionality and appearance of the websites delivering ICBT always include some public web pages and often closed pages requiring password (**Fig. 1** for a screenshot from a program). When there is interaction between a client and a clinician, more security is called for; email contact should be contained in a secure online environment, resembling Internet banking, with encrypted communication and a double-authentication procedure at login. The actual content of the treatment programs is often based on established CBT models, but increasingly also newer approaches that may not have been tested in face-to-face controlled trials. A typical ICBT program for anxiety and mood disorders may contain 8 to 15 treatment modules (sometimes referred to as lessons) and a structure that is similar to manual-based CBT. A treatment needs to start with psychoeducation and a rationale, and end with a closure and advice on how to handle setbacks. In between, typical CBT components are presented such as diary keeping, behavioral activation, exposure exercises, cognitive restructuring, relaxation, and a range of other techniques and procedures that are presented in text, as streamed video, in sound files, and increasingly with a presentation format that is responsive to where the web site is presented. Because many clients access the Internet via their phones, systems need to be sensitive to where the clients view their treatment (eg, on a smartphone, computer, or tablet). There are also specific smartphone apps that are developed and used as adjuncts to ICBT,[14] but also as a separate treatment format.[15] Two additional forms of Internet treatment should be mentioned also, with one being bias modification training[16] and the other use of virtual reality programs.[17] We do not comment further on these 2 approaches in this article, because they belong to a different category of treatments than regular ICBT.

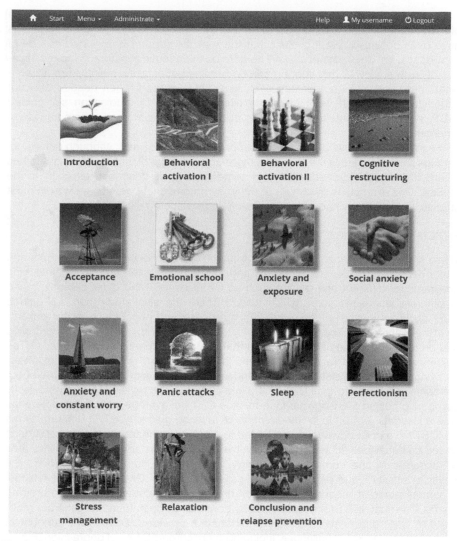

Fig. 1. Screenshot from a tailored Internet-based cognitive–behavioral therapy for depression program.

Homework is a common feature of ICBT programs. Feedback on homework completion can be automated, but more commonly personal when the treatment is guided by a clinician. This is an important distinction in that previously there was a clear indication that unguided programs led to more dropout and were less effective,[18] which was confirmed in a more recent review.[19] There are, however, exceptions where there is at least some form of initial clinical contact between the client and the researchers/clinicians, and in a review on depression studies a linear association between amount contact and outcome was found.[20] Programs have been improved and unguided programs with automated features have recently been found to generate large effects and minimal dropout.[21]

The role of the supporting clinician has generated publications investigating the role of therapeutic alliance,[22] therapist,[23] and client[24] behavior. Overall, small correlations have been observed, but it is clear that the way the support is provided can be of importance, but does not necessarily need to be therapeutic in nature.[25] Indeed, a series of studies showed that support can be provided effectively, mainly from a "technical" perspective.[26] Another approach is to offer support when needed and not scheduled, which can work for some client groups.[27] In studies on self-guided ICBT, it is often possible for the client to contact the clinician/researchers in case of emergency.[28]

In sum, there are several overlapping approaches to ICBT and, although consistent findings have emerged in the literature, there are examples of differences in outcomes given differences in procedures that may not always be described explicitly in the studies. One example is treatment of panic symptoms that has worked well in most studies, but in 1 study had an unexpectedly high dropout rate.[29]

EFFECTS ON DEPRESSION

There are a large number of controlled trials on ICBT for depressive symptoms and major depression.[30] Several programs and approaches have been tested, including programs for different age groups such as adolescents[31] and older persons,[32] and in different languages such as Chinese.[33] There are also studies on self-guided ICBT showing small (Hedges $g = 0.27$), but consistent, effects in a recent patient-level meta-analysis.[34] The format allows for large trials and in 1 randomized, controlled trial on a program called Deprexis more than 1013 participants were included.[35] The evidence with regard to clinician-guided ICBT has been reviewed several times, showing large and consistent results.[36] Indeed, effect sizes for guided ICBT are about the same as for face-to-face CBT,[37] and in a meta-analytic review of 5 studies directly comparing guided ICBT against face-to-face CBT the average, effect size difference was a Hedge's g of 0.12, in the direction of favoring guided ICBT.[38] Different forms on ICBT have been developed and tested in addition to the more standard approach based on behavioral activation and cognitive therapy,[39] including programs informed by acceptance and commitment therapy,[40,41] but also non-CBT approaches like physical activity[42] and psychodynamic psychotherapy.[43] Given the risk of relapse, programs aimed at secondary prevention have been developed and show promising results.[44] In sum, ICBT for depression has consistently been found to generate moderate to large effects when clinician guidance is provided. Despite the amount of research, there remain challenges, including more chronic forms of depression and bipolar disorders.

EFFECTS ON ANXIETY

Programs and controlled trials are available for most anxiety disorders, including different age groups, even if a majority of trials have been on adults. There is 1 Cochrane review on ICBT for anxiety disorders concluding that ICBT is effective,[45] with a standardized mean difference against no treatment control of −1.06, which is a large effect. They also concluded that therapist-guided ICBT potentially is as effective as face-to-face CBT. Here, we list conditions for which ICBT has been evaluated and also cite comparative studies answering the question if ICBT is equally effective as face-to-face CBT. In terms of treatment components, most studies and programs include psychoeducation, exposure, and cognitive techniques.[2]

Specific phobia has not been studied extensively, and 2 small controlled trials indicated that guided ICBT was effective, but not as effective as single-session exposure treatment on behavioral measures.[46,47] Other studies have included clients with phobia[48,49] and in 1 pilot study children aged 8 to 12 years were found to benefit from ICBT.[50]

Panic disorder and panic attacks have been the topic of several ICBT studies, including 3 comparative studies showing that guided ICBT can be as effective as face-to-face CBT.[51–53] Studies have also been conducted in more regular clinical settings (effectiveness) suggesting, that it is possible to transfer the treatment into regular care.[54] Clients with panic attacks and panic disorder have also been included in studies on transdiagnostic[55] and tailored ICBT.[56] Overall, effect sizes against no treatment control have been moderate to large across these trials and in the direct comparisons minor differences have been observed.

There are a few controlled studies on ICBT for generalized anxiety disorder showing positive results including long-term follow-up 3 years after treatment completion.[57] There are, however, to our knowledge no comparative trials against face-to-face CBT. Although there is 1 study on ICBT influenced by acceptance and commitment therapy,[58] with moderate to large between-group effects on symptoms of generalized anxiety disorder (Cohen's $d = 0.70$ to 0.98), most recent studies have been on transdiagnostic[21] and tailored ICBT in which participants with generalized anxiety disorder have been included.[59]

Social anxiety disorder is probably the condition, with the exception of depression, that has been studied in most controlled ICBT trials, beginning with the first study from Sweden.[60] There are 3 published studies comparing guided ICBT against face-to-face CBT showing similar outcomes[61–63] and also studies on long-term effects[64] and effectiveness in regular clinical settings.[65] This condition stands out because there are at least 5 different research groups who have found similar effects of ICBT and a study conducted in Romania with a program that was translated and culturally adapted from the Swedish ICBT program for social anxiety disorder.[66] Effects tend to be moderate to large, with the Romanian study having a between-group effect size of $d = 1.19$ on symptoms of social anxiety disorder. This finding highlights the possibility to rapidly disseminate findings across languages and borders, which has been more difficult with regular psychotherapy given needs to provide training and supervision.

When it comes to posttraumatic stress disorder and symptoms of posttraumatic stress, the first controlled trial was on a Dutch program called Interapy.[67] There have been several subsequent trials and, in a meta-analysis of ICBT for posttraumatic stress disorder, medium to large between-group effects were found based on 20 studies.[68] There are also studies conducted in different setting and languages, including war-traumatized Arab patients[69] and women who have experienced a traumatic childbirth.[70] We are not aware of any direct comparisons against face-to-face CBT, and posttraumatic stress disorder has to a lesser extent been part of transdiagnostic and tailored ICBT.

There have been few controlled studies on obsessive–compulsive disorder, but they indicate that ICBT with therapist guidance is effective,[71] with a between-group effect of $d = 0.85$. In an interesting study, ICBT was combined with D-cycloserine and, even if the medication did not show any overall benefit, post hoc analyses revealed that antidepressants significantly impaired treatment response in the D-cycloserine group but not the placebo group.[72] There are to date no direct comparisons against face-to-face CBT and no effectiveness studies conducted in regular clinical settings.

There is only 1 published controlled trial on body dysmorphic disorder. In the trial, 94 individuals with body dysmorphic disorder were randomized to either 12 weeks of guided ICBT with 8 modules or to online supportive therapy for 12 weeks.[73] Results at posttreatment showed a between-group effect size of $d = 0.97$ on the main outcome measure (Yale-Brown obsessive compulsive scale for body dysmorphic disorder).

Apart from the studies and programs for specific anxiety and obsessive–compulsive disorder–related disorders, there are several controlled trials on transdiagnostic and tailored ICBT.[59] This is a way to handle the issue of comorbidity between disorders and problems. Briefly, transdiagnostic ICBT covers shared techniques used in the treatment across disorders (eg, exposure) and tailored ICBT instead adapts treatment according to patient profile and preferred treatment targets (eg, stress problems). In a meta-analysis of 19 randomized trials, the controlled effect size for ICBT on anxiety and depression outcomes was medium to large (anxiety, $g = 0.82$; depression, $g = 0.79$).[59] There are no indications that these 2 approaches are less effective when compared against disorder-specific ICBT.[74]

In sum, clinician-guided ICBT for anxiety disorders seems to be effective, but there are still few direct comparisons against face-to-face CBT and some conditions, like obsessive–compulsive disorder, for which there are few studies.

MODERATORS AND MEDIATORS

In parallel with the controlled trials studies on predictors, moderators and mediators of outcome in ICBT have been published. Although there are clinical observations on what makes ICBT work,[75] the empirical literature is inconsistent with few if any robust predictors and moderators observed. For example, cognitive function,[76] genetics, age, and socioeconomic status have not been consistently associated with outcome,[77] and there are still few studies on mediators of outcome. It is important to note a lack of good theories specific for the treatment format; most studies have focused on either client factors, the therapeutic relationship, or disorder-specific mechanisms.[1] Factors such as adherence and treatment credibility have been studied and associations between credibility, module completion, and subsequent treatment outcome have been observed.[78] Interestingly, adherence in guided ICBT does not seem to be worse than in face-to-face CBT,[79] which is important to note, because Internet interventions with no therapist contact are known to be associated with poor adherence and high dropout in many studies.

DISCUSSION

In this brief article, we have covered a large number of studies in the field of psychiatry and concluded that clinician-guided ICBT seems to work as well as face-to-face CBT for some disorders. ICBT has been found to be effective for somatic conditions as well, for example, tinnitus and irritable bowel syndrome.[1] One possibility, yet to be explored, is to combine treatments for somatic and psychological problems. This has to some extent been done in tailored ICBT with, for example, treatment modules for insomnia when treating depression,[80] but there is room for further additions because comorbidity is substantial, in particular among primary care patients and older persons.

Research in this area can develop in different ways and one promising possibility is to include brain imaging techniques in treatment studies, which may generate strong predictions by means of machine learning approaches.[81] Machine learning could potentially also be used in the search for outcome predictors using behavioral data. Another development that is to be explored is to view ICBT as partly patient education and to test knowledge acquisition after treatment.[82] Because psychoeducation plays a major role in CBT the actual role of learning and what clients recall from their treatment is not clearly established. Given the large samples in ICBT trials and the fact that interventions are clearly defined and stay the same across clients (in contrast with face-to-face treatments, where the therapist may drift), it is possible to generate new knowledge about mechanisms of change, including the role of knowledge. Another development is to focus on problems that people have, not seldom of transdiagnostic nature, instead of diagnoses. One such example is a treatment for procrastination that was found to be effective.[83] Over the years, new knowledge has emerged regarding the cost effectiveness of ICBT with the predicted conclusion that it is cost effective,[84] and also a series of studies on the negative effects of treatment, which are relatively rare but can occur.[85] In addition to quantitative studies, there is also much to be learned from open-ended qualitative studies; for example, in 1 study that showed that some clients in ICBT may go through the treatment without engaging.[86]

There are additional limitations of ICBT apart from the possibility of negative effects for some clients. First, most programs require a certain reading level, because instructions are provided mostly in text. Second, in many studies participants have tended to be fairly well-educated, which may not be different from typical psychotherapy studies but still limits the possibility to generalize findings to regular medical settings. Third, even if direct comparative studies against face-to-face CBT show minor differences in outcome, it is still the case the few studies have used credible attention control conditions, which raises questions regarding the specificity of the findings.

Despite these limitations, the research and clinical implementation studies are promising and may result in increased access to evidence-based psychological treatment. Many questions remain to be answered, but given that information technology is likely here to stay for a while, it is our belief that clinicians will increasingly blend their regular services with ICBT either, as a complement or as an alternative for some clients.

REFERENCES

1. Andersson G. Internet-delivered psychological treatments. Annu Rev Clin Psychol 2016;12:157–79.

2. Andersson G. The internet and CBT: a clinical guide. Boca Raton (FL): CRC Press; 2015.

3. van Ballegooijen W, Riper H, Cuijpers P, et al. Validation of online psychometric instruments for common mental health disorders: a systematic review. BMC Psychiatry 2016;16:45.

4. Mohr DC, Burns MN, Schueller SM, et al. Behavioral intervention technologies: evidence review and recommendations for future research in mental health. Gen Hosp Psychiatry 2013;35:332–8.

5. Sholomskas DE, Syracuse-Siewert G, Rounsaville BJ, et al. We don't train in vain: a dissemination trial of three strategies of training clinicians in cognitive-behavioral therapy. J Consult Clin Psychol 2005;73:106–15.

6. Rakovshik SG, McManus F, Vazquez-Montes M, et al. Is supervision necessary? Examining the effects of internet-based CBT training with and without supervision. J Consult Clin Psychol 2016;84(3):191–9.

7. Andersson G, Carlbring P, Lindefors N. History and current status of ICBT. In: Lindefors N, Andersson G, editors. Guided internet-based treatments in psychiatry. Switzerland: Springer; 2016. p. 1–16.

8. Marks IM, Shaw S, Parkin R. Computer-assisted treatments of mental health problems. Clin Psychol Sci Prac 1998;5:51–170.

9. Marrs RW. A meta-analysis of bibliotherapy studies. Am J Community Psychol 1995;23:843–70.
10. Keeley H, Williams C, Shapiro DA. A United Kingdom survey of accredited cognitive behaviour therapists' attitudes towards and use of structured self-help materials. Behav Cognit Psychother 2002;30:193–203.
11. Andersson G, Bergström J, Buhrman M, et al. Development of a new approach to guided self-help via the internet. The Swedish experience. J Technol Hum Serv 2008;26:161–81.
12. Vlaescu G, Alasjö A, Miloff A, et al. Features and functionality of the Iterapi platform for internet-based psychological treatment. Internet Interv 2016;6:107–14.
13. Bennett K, Bennett AJ, Griffiths KM. Security considerations for e-mental health interventions. J Med Internet Res 2010;12(5):e61.
14. Ivanova E, Lindner P, Ly KH, et al. Guided and unguided acceptance and commitment therapy for social anxiety disorder and/or panic disorder provided via the internet and a smartphone application: a randomized controlled trial. J Anxiety Disord 2016;44:27–35.
15. Ly KH, Trüschel A, Jarl L, et al. Behavioral activation vs. mindfulness-based guided self-help treatment administered through a smartphone application: a randomized controlled trial. BMJ Open 2014;4:e003440.
16. Carlbring P, Apelstrand M, Sehlin H, et al. Internet-delivered attention training in individuals with social anxiety disorder - a double blind randomized controlled trial. BMC Psychiatry 2012;12:66.
17. Lindner P, Miloff A, Hamilton W, et al. Creating state of the art, next-generation virtual reality exposure therapies for anxiety disorders using consumer hardware platforms: design considerations and future direction. Cogn Behav Ther 2017; 46(5):404–20.
18. Andersson G, Cuijpers P. Internet-based and other computerized psychological treatments for adult depression: a meta-analysis. Cogn Behav Ther 2009;38: 196–205.
19. Baumeister H, Reichler L, Munzinger M, et al. The impact of guidance on internet-based mental health interventions - a systematic review. Internet Interv 2014;1: 205–15.
20. Johansson R, Andersson G. Internet-based psychological treatments for depression. Expert Rev Neurother 2012;12:861–70.
21. Dear BF, Staples LG, Terides MD, et al. Transdiagnostic versus disorder-specific and clinician-guided versus self-guided internet-delivered treatment for generalized anxiety disorder and comorbid disorders: a randomized controlled trial. J Anxiety Disord 2015;36:63–77.
22. Andersson G, Paxling B, Wiwe M, et al. Therapeutic alliance in guided Internet-delivered cognitive behavioral treatment of depression, generalized anxiety disorder and social anxiety disorder. Behav Res Ther 2012;50:544–50.
23. Holländare F, Gustafsson SA, Berglind M, et al. Therapist behaviours in internet-based cognitive behaviour therapy (ICBT) for depressive symptoms. Internet Interv 2016;3:1–7.
24. Svartvatten N, Segerlund M, Dennhag I, et al. A content analysis of client e-mails in guided internet-based cognitive behavior therapy for depression. Internet Interv 2015;2:121–7.
25. Sanchez-Ortiz VC, Munro C, Startup H, et al. The role of email guidance in internet-based cognitive-behavioural self-care treatment for bulimia nervosa. Eur Eat Disord Rev 2011;19:342–8.

26. Titov N, Andrews G, Davies M, et al. Internet treatment for depression: a randomized controlled trial comparing clinician vs. technician assistance. PLoS One 2010;5:e10939.
27. Rheker J, Andersson G, Weise C. The role of "on demand" therapist guidance vs. no support in the treatment of tinnitus via the internet: a randomized controlled trial. Internet Interv 2015;2:189–99.
28. Titov N, Dear BF, Staples L, et al. The first 30 months of the MindSpot Clinic: evaluation of a national e-mental health service against project objectives. Aust N Z J Psychiatry 2016. [Epub ahead of print].
29. van Ballegooijen W, Riper H, Klein B, et al. An Internet-based guided self-help intervention for panic symptoms: randomized controlled trial. J Med Internet Res 2013;15(7):e154.
30. Andersson G, Wagner B, Cuijpers P. ICBT for depression. In: Lindefors N, Andersson G, editors. Guided internet-based treatments in psychiatry. Switzerland: Springer; 2016. p. 17–32.
31. Ebert DD, Zarski AC, Christensen H, et al. Internet and computer-based cognitive behavioral therapy for anxiety and depression in youth: a meta-analysis of randomized controlled outcome trials. PLoS One 2015;10(3):e0119895.
32. Titov N, Dear BF, Ali S, et al. Clinical and cost-effectiveness of therapist-guided internet-delivered cognitive behavior therapy for older adults with symptoms of depression: a randomized controlled trial. Behav Ther 2015;46:193–205.
33. Choi I, Zou J, Titov N, et al. Culturally attuned internet treatment for depression amongst Chinese Australians: a randomised controlled trial. J Affect Disord 2012;136:459–68.
34. Karyotaki E, Riper H, Twisk J, et al. Efficacy of self-guided internet-based cognitive behavioral therapy in the treatment of depressive symptoms: a meta-analysis of individual participant data. JAMA Psychiatry 2017;74(4):351–9.
35. Klein JP, Berger T, Schröder J, et al. Effects of a psychological internet intervention in the treatment of mild to moderate depressive symptoms: results of the EVIDENT study, a randomised controlled trial. Psychother Psychosom 2016;85:218–28.
36. Richards D, Richardson T. Computer-based psychological treatments for depression: a systematic review and meta-analysis. Clin Psychol Rev 2012;32:329–42.
37. Cuijpers P, Riper H, Andersson G. Internet-based treatment of depression. Curr Opin Psychol 2015;4:131–5.
38. Andersson G, Topooco N, Havik OE, et al. Internet-supported versus face-to-face cognitive behavior therapy for depression. Expert Rev Neurother 2016;16:55–60.
39. Andersson G, Bergström J, Holländare F, et al. Internet-based self-help for depression: a randomised controlled trial. Br J Psychiatry 2005;187:456–61.
40. Lappalainen P, Granlund A, Siltanen S, et al. ACT internet-based vs face-to-face? a randomized controlled trial of two ways to deliver acceptance and commitment therapy for depressive symptoms: an 18-month follow-up. Behav Res Ther 2014;61:43–54.
41. Carlbring P, Hägglund M, Luthström A, et al. Internet-based behavioral activation and acceptance-based treatment for depression: a randomized controlled trial. J Affect Disord 2013;148:331–7.
42. Ström M, Uckelstam C-J, Andersson G, et al. Internet-delivered therapist-guided physical activity for mild to moderate depression: a randomized controlled trial. Peer J 2013;1:e178.

43. Johansson R, Ekbladh S, Hebert A, et al. Psychodynamic guided self-help for adult depression through the internet: a randomised controlled trial. PLoS One 2012;7(5):e38021.

44. Holländare F, Johnsson S, Randestad M, et al. Randomized trial of internet-based relapse prevention for partially remitted depression. Acta Psychiatr Scand 2011; 124:285–94.

45. Olthuis JV, Watt MC, Bailey K, et al. Therapist-supported Internet cognitive behavioural therapy for anxiety disorders in adults. Cochrane Database Syst Rev 2015;(3):CD011565.

46. Andersson G, Waara J, Jonsson U, et al. Internet-based vs. one-session exposure treatment of snake phobia: a randomized controlled trial. Cogn Behav Ther 2013;42:284–91.

47. Andersson G, Waara J, Jonsson U, et al. Internet-based self-help vs. one-session exposure in the treatment of spider phobia: a randomized controlled trial. Cogn Behav Ther 2009;38:114–20.

48. Vigerland S, Ljótsson B, Thulin U, et al. Internet-delivered cognitive behavioral therapy for children with anxiety disorders: a randomized controlled trial. Behav Res Ther 2016;76:47–56.

49. Kok RN, van Straten A, Beekman AT, et al. Short-term effectiveness of web-based guided self-help for phobic outpatients: randomized controlled trial. J Med Internet Res 2014;16:e226.

50. Vigerland S, Thulin U, Svirsky L, et al. Internet-delivered CBT for children with specific phobia: a pilot study. Cogn Behav Ther 2013;42:303–14.

51. Bergström J, Andersson G, Ljótsson B, et al. Internet- versus group-administered cognitive behaviour therapy for panic disorder in a psychiatric setting: a randomised trial. BMC Psychiatry 2010;10:54.

52. Kiropoulos LA, Klein B, Austin DW, et al. Is internet-based CBT for panic disorder and agoraphobia as effective as face-to-face CBT? J Anxiety Disord 2008;22: 1273–84.

53. Carlbring P, Nilsson-Ihrfelt E, Waara J, et al. Treatment of panic disorder: live therapy vs. self-help via internet. Behav Res Ther 2005;43:1321–33.

54. Hedman E, Ljótsson B, Rück C, et al. Effectiveness of internet-based cognitive behaviour therapy for panic disorder in routine psychiatric care. Acta Psychiatr Scand 2013;128:457–67.

55. Johnston L, Titov N, Andrews G, et al. A RCT of a transdiagnostic internet-delivered treatment for three anxiety disorders: examination of support roles and disorder-specific outcomes. PLoS One 2011;6:e28079.

56. Silfvernagel K, Carlbring P, Kabo J, et al. Individually tailored internet-based treatment of young adults and adults with panic symptoms: a randomized controlled trial. J Med Internet Res 2012;14(3):e65.

57. Paxling B, Almlöv J, Dahlin M, et al. Guided internet-delivered cognitive behavior therapy for generalized anxiety disorder: a randomized controlled trial. Cogn Behav Ther 2011;40:159–73.

58. Dahlin M, Ryberg M, Vernmark K, et al. Internet-delivered acceptance-based behavior therapy for generalized anxiety disorder: a pilot study. Internet Interv 2016;6:16–21.

59. Păsărelu C, Andersson G, Bergman Nordgren L, et al. Internet-delivered transdiagnostic and tailored cognitive behavioral therapy for anxiety and depression: a systematic review and meta-analysis. Cogn Behav Ther 2017;46:1–28.

60. Andersson G, Carlbring P, Holmström A, et al. Internet-based self-help with therapist feedback and in-vivo group exposure for social phobia: a randomized controlled trial. J Consult Clin Psychol 2006;74:677–86.
61. Hedman E, Andersson G, Ljótsson B, et al. Internet-based cognitive behavior therapy vs. cognitive behavioral group therapy for social anxiety disorder: a randomized controlled non-inferiority trial. PLoS One 2011;6(3):e18001.
62. Andrews G, Davies M, Titov N. Effectiveness randomized controlled trial of face to face versus internet cognitive behaviour therapy for social phobia. Aust N Z J Psychiatry 2011;45:337–40.
63. Andrews G, Cuijpers P, Craske MG, et al. Computer therapy for the anxiety and depressive disorders is effective, acceptable and practical health care: a meta-analysis. PLoS One 2010;5:e13196.
64. Hedman E, Furmark T, Carlbring P, et al. Five-year follow-up of internet-based cognitive behaviour therapy for social anxiety disorder. J Med Internet Res 2011;13(2):e39.
65. El Alaoui S, Hedman E, Kaldo V, et al. Effectiveness of internet-based cognitive behavior therapy for social anxiety disorder in clinical psychiatry. J Consult Clin Psychol 2015;83:902–14.
66. Tulbure BT, Szentagotai A, David O, et al. Internet-delivered cognitive-behavioral therapy for social anxiety disorder in Romania: a randomized controlled trial. PLoS One 2015;10:e0123997.
67. Lange A, Rietdijk D, Hudcovicova M, et al. Interapy: a controlled randomized trial of the standardized treatment of posttraumatic stress through the Internet. J Consult Clin Psychol 2003;71:901–9.
68. Kuester A, Niemeyer H, Knaevelsrud C. Internet-based interventions for posttraumatic stress: a meta-analysis of randomized controlled trials. Clin Psychol Rev 2016;43:1–16.
69. Knaevelsrud C, Brand J, Lange A, et al. Web-based psychotherapy for posttraumatic stress disorder in war-traumatized Arab patients: randomized controlled trial. J Med Internet Res 2015;17:e71.
70. Nieminen K, Berg I, Frankenstein K, et al. Internet-delivered cognitive behaviour therapy of posttraumatic stress symptoms following childbirth - a randomized controlled trial. Cogn Behav Ther 2016;45:287–306.
71. Pozza A, Andersson G, Dèttore D. Therapist-guided internet-based cognitive-behavioural therapy for adult obsessive-compulsive disorder: a meta-analysis. Eur Psychiatry 2016;33(Supplement):S276–7.
72. Andersson E, Hedman E, Enander J, et al. D-cycloserine vs placebo as adjunct to cognitive behavioral therapy for obsessive-compulsive disorder and interaction with antidepressants: a randomized clinical trial. JAMA Psychiatry 2015;72:659–67.
73. Enander J, Andersson E, Mataix-Cols D, et al. Therapist guided internet based cognitive behavioural therapy for body dysmorphic disorder: single blind randomised controlled trial. BMJ 2016;352:i241.
74. Berger T, Boettcher J, Caspar F. Internet-based guided self-help for several anxiety disorders: a randomized controlled trial comparing a tailored with a standardized disorder-specific approach. Psychotherapy 2014;51:207–19.
75. Andersson G, Carlbring P, Berger T, et al. What makes internet therapy work? Cogn Behav Ther 2009;38(S1):55–60.
76. Lindner P, Carlbring P, Flodman E, et al. Does cognitive flexibility predict treatment gains in internet-delivered psychological treatment of social anxiety disorder, depression, or tinnitus? Peer J 2016;4:e1934.

77. Hedman E, Andersson E, Ljótsson B, et al. Clinical and genetic outcome determinants of internet- and group-based cognitive behavior therapy for social anxiety disorder. Acta Psychiatr Scand 2012;126:126–36.
78. Hedman E, Andersson E, Lekander M, et al. Predictors in internet-delivered cognitive behavior therapy and behavioral stress management for severe health anxiety. Behav Res Ther 2015;64:49–55.
79. van Ballegooijen W, Cuijpers P, van Straten A, et al. Adherence to internet-based and face-to-face cognitive behavioural therapy for depression: a meta-analysis. PLoS One 2014;9:e100674.
80. Johansson R, Sjöberg E, Sjögren M, et al. Tailored vs. standardized internet-based cognitive behavior therapy for depression and comorbid symptoms: a randomized controlled trial. PLoS One 2012;7(5):e36905.
81. Månsson KNT, Frick A, Boraxbekk C-J, et al. Predicting long-term outcome of Internet-delivered cognitive behavior therapy for social anxiety disorder using fMRI and support vector machine learning. Transl Psychiatry 2015;5:e530.
82. Andersson G, Carlbring P, Furmark T, on behalf of the SOFIE Research Group. Therapist experience and knowledge acquisition in internet-delivered CBT for social anxiety disorder: a randomized controlled trial. PLoS One 2012;7(5):e37411.
83. Rozental A, Forsell E, Svensson A, et al. Internet-based cognitive behavior therapy for procrastination: a randomized controlled trial. J Consult Clin Psychol 2015;83:808–24.
84. Donker T, Blankers M, Hedman E, et al. Economic evaluations of internet interventions for mental health: a systematic review. Psychol Med 2015;45:3357–76.
85. Rozental A, Magnusson K, Boettcher J, et al. For better or worse: an individual patient data meta-analysis of deterioration among participants receiving internet-based cognitive behavior therapy. J Consult Clin Psychol 2016;85:160–77.
86. Bendelin N, Hesser H, Dahl J, et al. Experiences of guided internet-based cognitive-behavioural treatment for depression: a qualitative study. BMC Psychiatry 2011;11:107.

Cultural Adaptations of Cognitive Behavioral Therapy

Devon E. Hinton, MD, PhD[a],*, Anushka Patel, MA[b]

KEYWORDS

- Culture • CBT • Cultural adaptation • Refugees • Minority populations

KEY POINTS

- In increasingly multicultural societies, cognitive behavioral therapy (CBT) must be made appropriate for diverse groups.
- This article examines cultural adaptations of CBT, focusing on anxiety and depressive disorders.
- The article presents a culturally informed transdiagnostic model of how anxious-depressive distress is generated and culturally shaped.
- Guided by this model, it discusses how interventions can be designed to decrease anxiety-type and depressive-type psychopathology in a culturally sensitive way.
- It describes such concepts as explanatory model bridging, cultural grounding, and contextual sensitivity.

INTRODUCTION

Evidence demonstrates that cognitive behavioral therapy (CBT) is effective for a wide range of disorders, including posttraumatic stress disorder (PTSD[1]). However, most research on CBT has focused on Western populations and research is just beginning to examine whether CBT is effective for ethnic minority and refugee groups, and for other global contexts, and how CBT should be adapted in such cases.[2–9] A systematic review of 10 randomized controlled trials on treatment of refugees with mental health problems found some promise in CBT and argued that there is a need for adapting treatments to the local cultural context.[10] Another review of 76 studies on culturally adapted (CA) mental health interventions for a wide range of disorders found that interventions targeted to specific ethnic groups produced 4 times stronger effects than those provided to diverse ethnic groups.[11] Yet another review confirmed that CA

[a] Department of Psychiatry, Massachusetts General Hospital, Harvard Medical School, 15 Parkman Street, WACC 812, Boston, MA 02114, USA; [b] Department of Psychology, The University of Tulsa, 800 South Tucker Drive, Tulsa, OK 74104, USA
* Corresponding author.
E-mail address: devon_hinton@hms.harvard.edu

Psychiatr Clin N Am 40 (2017) 701–714
http://dx.doi.org/10.1016/j.psc.2017.08.006
0193-953X/17/© 2017 Elsevier Inc. All rights reserved.

treatment is more effective than unadapted treatment ($d = .32$) in a direct-comparison meta-analysis, and found that making the explanatory model consonant with that of the patient is particularly important.[12]

How can CBT treatments be CA? Bernal and colleagues[13(p362)] define cultural adaptation as the "systematic modification of an evidence-based treatment to account for language, culture, and context in a way that is consistent with the client's cultural patterns, meanings and values." CBT can be CA in several ways. Examples include: standard CBT techniques may need particular explanation and framing, specific local catastrophic cognitions may need to be modified, CBT techniques may need to be made more tolerable (especially among groups with excessive arousal), certain types of psychopathology (eg, somatic symptoms, panic, and arousal) may need to be especially targeted, and local types of stigma may need to be addressed.

To know how to intervene in a culturally sensitive way with anxiety and depressive disorders, it is first necessary to develop an understanding of how culture shapes anxiety-type and depressive-type distress in different cultural populations. Culture powerfully influences the way in which anxiety and depression are generated, experienced, and treated.[14–16] **Fig. 1** presents a general model of how episodes of anxiety-type and depressive-type distress are generated and how culture plays a key role. The processes outlined in this model can be addressed in various ways based on CBT principles.

Table 1 outlines some of the interventions that can be used to affect the processes outlined in **Fig. 1** and how those interventions can be CA. Among the interventions, addressing a patient's explanatory model is a key aspect.[12] The explanatory model is the way in which a group understands an illness experience, including ideas about causation, key symptoms, and cures.[17] Many of the interventions in **Table 1** involve addressing and modifying the patient's model of the disorder they have. Understanding the client's interpretation of symptoms and providing treatment congruent with their explanatory model is a key ingredient in CA treatment, which may be called explanatory model bridging (**Fig. 2**). See later discussion for illustration of several of the principles outlined in **Table 1**, with examples of cultural adaptation, in particular from the first author's treatment: CA-CBT for trauma-related disorder.[18–24] In this article we attempt to illustrate how to culturally ground CBT, to make CBT more contextually sensitive.

CULTURAL ADAPTATIONS OF COGNITIVE BEHAVIORAL THERAPY
Creating Positive Expectancy and Treatment Credibility in a Culturally Appropriate Way

Positive expectancy greatly increases positive outcomes in therapy.[25] Positive expectancy results when patients believe that the treatment will improve the problems that are of most concern to them. It has 2 aspects: that patients believe that the treatment addresses the problems of concern to them and that patients believe that the treatment is capable of reducing those problems. To create positive expectancy, the clinician must know what patients think their problem is.[26,27] For example, Japanese individuals with social phobia may consider *taijin kyofusho*, with symptoms such as fearing one's odor is offending others, rather than "social phobia" as their key concern. A Cambodian individual may see a so-called weak heart, dizziness, sleep paralysis, dizziness, and nightmares as the key problems rather than PTSD, a concept about which they have little familiarity. If one informs the patient that the treatment will address the problems of concern to him or her,

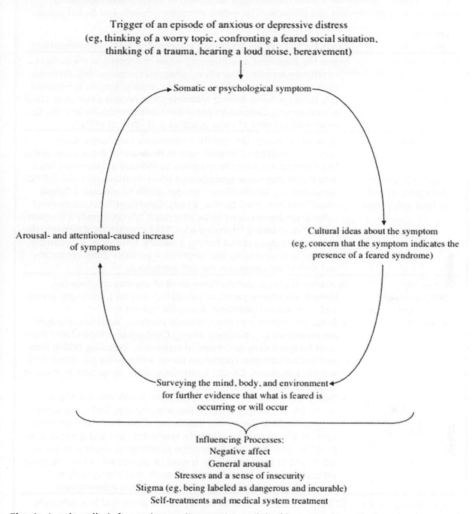

Trigger of an episode of anxious or depressive distress
(eg, thinking of a worry topic, confronting a feared social situation,
thinking of a trauma, hearing a loud noise, bereavement)

Somatic or psychological symptom

Arousal- and attentional-caused increase
of symptoms

Cultural ideas about the symptom
(eg, concern that the symptom indicates the
presence of a feared syndrome)

Surveying the mind, body, and environment
for further evidence that what is feared is
occurring or will occur

Influencing Processes:
Negative affect
General arousal
Stresses and a sense of insecurity
Stigma (eg, being labeled as dangerous and incurable)
Self-treatments and medical system treatment

Fig. 1. A culturally informed transdiagnostic model of how psychopathology is generated.

specifically naming the problems of concern, positive expectancy is greatly increased.

As a key way to positive expectancy, treatment studies in cross-cultural settings should include a list of locally salient complaints, such as key somatic complaints, and should include a list of cultural syndromes. The clinician should specifically state that the treatment will address those complaints. We call this a symptom and syndrome addendum (SSA); for example, a Cambodian-SSA (C-SSA).[28,29] Certain locally salient complaints may be particularly important to assess across treatment: in some Latino groups, *ataques de nervios*,[19] and in Cambodian refugee groups, orthostatic dizziness (ie, dizziness on standing).[19,28–30] More generally, arousal symptoms can be listed and the patient told that those symptoms will be addressed. In treatment, queries can be given to elicit symptoms. (For other means of increasing positive expectancy, such as framing treatment using local analogies and comparing with local practices, see later discussion.)

Table 1
Ways to make cognitive behavioral therapy-type treatment of anxiety and depressive disorders more appropriate and efficacious for ethnic minority, refugee, and global groups

Treatment Intervention	Examples of How the Treatment Intervention Goal Is Accomplished
Create positive expectancy and treatment credibility	Frame the treatment as addressing issues of concern to the patient, which may include culturally emphasized symptoms (eg, dizziness, poor sleep, shortness of breath) and culturally specific syndromes (eg, *taijin kyofusho* among Japanese social phobia patients or *khyâl attacks* among Cambodian panic disorder patients). Present the CBT treatment in terms of local practices and ideas of efficacy.
Address locally salient catastrophic cognitions about symptoms, as well as local syndromes	In different cultures, the specific catastrophic cognitions about symptoms must be addressed, such as those about arousal symptoms (eg, Cambodians consider dizziness to indicate a dangerous *khyâl* attack that may cause syncope and other disasters) and about PTSD symptoms (eg, Cambodians consider startle to indicate a "weak heart" and imminent cardiac arrest). Catastrophic cognitions and cultural syndromes need to be addressed: transculturally a frequent cultural syndrome is "thinking a lot." The clinician must alleviate the patient's concerns about having a cultural syndrome, for example, explaining how anxiety and depression produce those symptoms and that those symptoms are not dangerous.
Address key dimensions of psychopathology in a group	In a cultural group, certain dimensions of psychopathology (eg, somatic symptoms, panic, or suicidality) may be particularly severe and need special attention. Examples include • Somatic symptoms: In many cultural contexts, somatic complaints are prominent (eg, dizziness among Cambodian refugees) and these must be specifically addressed in treatment, including taking into account catastrophic cognitions about and trauma associations to somatic sensations. CA-CBT addresses somatic symptoms in multiple ways (see **Table 2**). • Worry and generalized anxiety disorder (GAD): Uncontrollable worry drives multiple types of psychopathology, including somatic symptoms, GAD, panic, and depressive affect. Patients from other cultural groups may have specific worry domains and great severity of worry, and they may have great catastrophic cognitions about worry and its symptoms, which must be addressed, otherwise great arousal and psychopathology will result. Techniques such as meditation and applied stretching may be key interventions.
Use culturally specific metaphors, proverbs, stories, and analogies to convey CBT information and to create positive expectancy	CBT principles should be as far as possible presented in a culturally sensitive way, such as by using proverbs and expressions from the culture that express CBT principles. For example, to teach a Latino patient the effect of attentional focus on mood and the dangers of rumination, the phrase "Don't drown in a glass of water" (*no so ahoge en un vaso de agua*) can be used. CBT techniques may also be framed in terms of locally salient metaphors. These are other examples of the cultural grounding of CBT.
Present CBT information and techniques in terms of the local psychology, physiology, and spiritual tradition	Each culture will have certain ideas about how and why symptoms occur, which may be rooted in local religious traditions, such as Islam, Christianity, or Buddhism. The clinician should try to frame CBT information in terms of those local psychologies, physiologies, and religious traditions. For example, in Buddhism coldness is considered to be the ideal state, suggesting a centered mind unperturbed by worry, and so the CBT treatments can be presented as cooling and helping to center the mind. CBT-type techniques like mindfulness may have analogies in the local traditions. Framing treatment in terms of local explanatory models is a form of explanatory model bridging, a type of cultural grounding.

(*continued on next page*)

Table 1 *(continued)*	
Treatment Intervention	**Examples of How the Treatment Intervention Goal Is Accomplished**
Include CBT-consistent therapeutic techniques from the local traditions	Each culture will have certain methods to relieve distress. If possible, techniques from local traditions should be incorporated in the treatment (or at least the CBT techniques should be framed in terms of local religious traditions). Examples would be to include yoga for certain Indian populations, meditation and loving kindness for Buddhists, opening the Bible at random to read a passage or doing the rosary for certain Christian groups, or the practice of repeatedly saying the name of Allah (*dhikr*) for certain Islamic groups. Local proverbs and ethnopsychology also may be a therapeutic resource. CA-CBT elicits patient's self-treatments and encourages adaptive ones at the beginning of most sessions.
Promote a sense of self-esteem and self-efficacy in culturally appropriate way	Low self-esteem and self-efficacy drives psychopathology. It is important to create positive self-images that promote a positive self-image and a sense of self-efficacy. For example, in CA-CBT, for certain Asian groups, the image of the flexile wind-moved lotus is used as a positive self-image that promotes a sense of being able to adjust. Ending the CBT with culturally indicated transitional ritual may also change self-imagery.
Address stress and security issues	Living in a state of stress and insecurity has a major impact on psychopathology, such as increasing arousal and arousability. Every group will have particular sources of stress and insecurity and may have higher rates of certain types; for example, domestic abuse. Knowledge of these issues and teaching how to practically handle these issues is important, a problem-solving CBT. In addition, emotion regulation techniques need to be taught to reduce stress.
Adaptation of key CBT techniques to promote tolerability and cultural appropriateness	CBT techniques should be adapted as far as possible to each group. Examples include • Interoceptive exposure with reassociation: CA-CBT does interoceptive exposure with reassociation of somatic sensations to positive culturally appropriate imagery; when inducing dizziness in head rolling we have Latino patients think of the piñata game, a traditional game in which dizziness is induced. This is a much more tolerable means of interoceptive exposure. • Trauma exposure paired to the practice of emotion regulation: Patients from other cultural contexts may poorly tolerate traditional trauma exposure for several reasons, including high current stress. A phase approach is suggested and the use of novel techniques to make exposure more acceptable, such as immediately practicing emotion regulation techniques after exposure. This is done in CA-CBT.
Increase cognitive and emotion flexibility in a culturally appropriate way	Psychological flexibility is a key aspect of psychological health (eg, it promotes emotion regulation) and is a skill that is particularly important for refugees and minorities who need to negotiate between multiple cultural domains. Ideally culturally appropriate analogies and self-imagery should be taught to promote this skill; for example, local proverbs highlighting that skill. In CA-CBT, for example, muscle stretching is paired with cultural metaphors of flexibility.

(continued on next page)

Table 1 *(continued)*	
Treatment Intervention	**Examples of How the Treatment Intervention Goal Is Accomplished**
Reduce stigma	To reduce self-caused stigma, it is important to explain to patients that psychological disorders are treatable and to address local ideas about mental illness. Community-wide education may be needed. Treatment in primary care may reduce stigma.
End treatment with a culturally indicated transitional ritual	At the end of treatment, ideally, a culturally appropriate transition ritual is used. This creates a sense of positive expectancy about recovery. Also, these rituals often present a self-image and world-image that creates a sense of having recovered in respect to local religious and other cultural ideals, producing a more positive self-schema and world-schema.

Addressing Catastrophic Cognitions about Symptoms as well as Cultural Syndromes

Fig. 1 illustrates of the role of catastrophic cognitions in worsening anxiety and depressive disorders. Ideally, the clinician will be familiar with such fears in the local group and be able to specifically address them. We suggest that "thinking a lot," which is syndrome that occurs in some form in many cultures, can be investigated as an entrée into the local cultural context, that is, an introduction into the local conceptualizations of the mind, the body, and the spiritual tradition, and we have designed a survey instrument to do so.[31,32] Queries can also be included in treatment, such as asking what symptoms the person has and then asking what the fears about them are, which is what is done in CA-CBT. (In addition, in the CA-CBT manual, catastrophic cognitions about anxiety and PTSD symptoms for certain groups are specified; namely, for several Asian groups [Cambodian, Chinese, and Vietnamese] and for Latino populations.)

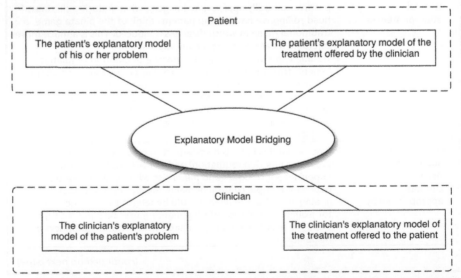

Fig. 2. The core clinical task of explanatory model bridging, with the clinical encounter configured as the negotiation of 4 types of explanatory models.

Anxiety and depressive symptoms are interpreted according to the local conceptualization of the mind, body, and the spiritual tradition. As examples of such fears, Cambodian patients often fear that dizziness, such as that induced by "thinking a lot," indicates the start of a *khyâl* attack; namely, a surge of *khyâl* substance upward in the body to cause various disasters[33]; and Latino patients fear that shakiness of the limbs or racing thoughts indicate a problem with *nervios* or an imminent *ataque de nervios*.[34–36] Or PTSD symptoms, from nightmares to startle, may give rise to such catastrophic cognitions. Many cultural groups fear that trauma recall indicates imminent insanity (eg, Cambodian refugees[37]), that trauma recall results from persecution by dangerous spirits of the dead, and that trauma-related nightmares and sleep paralysis are spiritual attacks (eg, Cambodian refugees and Rwandan trauma survivors).[38,39] Some groups consider startle to have the power to dislodge the soul and to cause death or serious illness (eg, Latino and Southeast Asian populations[35]). Some groups consider that startle indicates a dangerous weakness of the heart that brings about a general cardiac hyperreactivity that may lead to death (eg, Cambodian and Vietnamese refugees).[34]

Patients often attribute symptoms to a cultural syndrome, and this attribution may produce catastrophic cognitions that the symptoms indicate a serious bodily dysfunction, mental perturbation (eg, imminent insanity), and/or spiritual attack. These catastrophic cognitions start an escalating spiral of arousal, panic, somatic symptoms, and PTSD (see **Fig. 1**). Assessing cultural syndromes gives the clinician a better sense of the patient's experience of anxiety and depression, and the effect of anxiety and depression on his or her lifeworld and relationships. Knowledge of these syndromes allows the clinician to assess and modify key catastrophic cognitions. It also increases treatment adherence because some of the patient's key concerns are being addressed (for the clinical utility of assessing and treating cultural syndromes, see[34]).

As previously indicated, we have developed measures to examine cultural syndromes for these groups, such as the C-SSA.[29,40] The C-SSA aims to assess key somatic complaints and cultural syndromes found in the Cambodian group. The patient can be told that treatment addresses those symptoms and syndromes, which helps to decrease catastrophic cognitions and to create positive expectancy. The SSA also serves as a list of symptoms about which there are often catastrophic cognitions and cultural syndromes that need to be addressed. As examples of items in these SSAs, in our treatment of Cambodian populations, we specifically ask whether the patient fears having weak heart or *khyâl* attacks, how they treat episodes of those cultural syndromes, and what fears they have about them (for a review of these syndromes, see[35]). In our treatment of Latino patients, we specially assess and address in this same way key syndrome such syndromes as *nervios* and *ataque de nervios*.

Target Key Psychopathological Dimensions (eg, Somatic Symptoms)

In certain groups, some psychopathological dimensions may need particular therapeutic attention. Studies show that somatic complaints are particularly prominent among many non-English speakers.[41,42] **Fig. 1** illustrates how such somatic symptoms are produced, and we have discussed some of the ways these are addressed in a culturally sensitive way (eg, through addressing catastrophic cognitions). Other key means are interoceptive exposure with reassociation (see later discussion) and various means to decrease arousal, such as teaching emotion regulation, including somatic-focused emotion regulation, such as applied muscle relaxation and stretching.[43–45] In CA-CBT, somatic sensations are addressed in multiple ways (**Table 2**).

Table 2
How culturally adapted multiplex cognitive behavioral therapy reduces somatic symptoms

Treatment Goal	Examples of How the Treatment Goal Is Accomplished
Teaching how to relieve somatic symptoms through various techniques	• Applied muscle relaxation and applied stretching to reduce muscle tension, headache, and cold extremities • Training in diaphragmatic breathing to reduce chest tightness, dizziness, and cold extremities • Meditation training to teach to move attention away from somatic sensations
Modifying catastrophic cognitions about somatic sensations	• Education about how arousal causes somatic symptoms that are not dangerous • Addressing the patients' understanding of the symptoms and the dangers they pose, such as concerns that a somatic symptom indicates an imminent disaster like the onset of a cultural syndrome[46] • Interoceptive exposure and positive reassociation to somatic sensations (ie, traditional interoceptive exposure, such as head rotation or hyperventilation to induce dizziness, combined with creating positive associations to the induced symptom)
Reducing trauma associations to somatic sensations	• Education about the trauma associations to somatic symptoms • Exposure to trauma memories followed by practice of the trauma protocol • Interoceptive exposure and positive reassociation to trauma-related somatic sensations
Reducing conditioned fear responses to somatic sensations	• Interoceptive exposure to the somatic sensations and positive reassociations to those somatic sensations
Reducing triggers of somatic sensations	• Reduction of negative affectivity and general arousal through various techniques, such as somatic regulation techniques (eg, applied stretching) and emotion regulation techniques (eg, emotion labeling and distancing and the practice of loving kindness) • Reduction of disorders that generate somatic sensation such as worry or GAD (eg, through meditation), panic (eg, through addressing catastrophic cognitions and doing exposure), and PTSD (eg, through trauma recall exposure paired with emotion regulation practice)

Use Culturally Specific Proverbs, Stories, and Analogies to Convey Cognitive Behavioral Therapy Information and to Create Positive Expectancy

Proverbs and analogies can serve as adaptive cognitive sets to interpret reality that promote positive affect and serve as primers to adaptive functioning.[47–49] Proverbs and analogies can result in positive expectancy and alleviate negative affect, perhaps helping the individual to handle stress and negative emotions. They can be used to teach CBT information and may function as a form of emotion regulation. **Table 3** contains examples of proverbs. Using proverbs, cultural stories, and culturally appropriate analogies also helps to promote the patient's cultural self-esteem, that is, the patient's sense that he or she comes from a culture with a rich and important tradition of knowledge, which further decreases negative affect. Additionally, using proverbs, cultural stories, and culturally appropriate analogies can improve the therapeutic alliance; the patient feels the therapist understands and appreciates his or her cultural background.

Table 3 Examples of proverbs and culturally salient expressions that can be used therapeutically		
Group	Proverb or Culturally Salient Idiom	Therapeutic Meaning
Latino	"Don't drown in a glass of water" (*No se ahoge en un vaso de agua*)	Don't ruminate on an issue or problem to the point it causes you great distress.
Latino	"Undrown yourself" (*Desohogarse*)	Say what bothers you or you will drown in your unspoken distress (ie, in this idiom, an unspoken topic of distress is analogized to a drowning water).
Cambodian	"If you don't get angry 1 time, you gain 100 days of happiness" (*Gom kheung medoong baan sok merooy thngay*)	Realize the negative consequences of anger episodes in which the person says or does something that has long-term negative effects.
Cambodian	"Don't *reek* by yourself" (*reek* means "to carry the pole at the shoulder, with a weight balanced at either side")	Share with others your problems or you will become overburdened and overwhelmed.
African American	"Rebound"	You can rebound after a missed "shot"; that is, you can recover from a reversal or mistake if you engage and mobilize to recover.

For example, to teach Latino patients the importance of decentering and the negative spiral created by narrowly focusing on a negative cognition, one can use the proverb, "*No se ahoge en un vaso de agua*," meaning "Don't drown in a glass of water." This is an example of tapping into the local model of mind and traditional ways of handling distress enshrined in a proverb that teaches about the danger of attending too narrowly to a single subject or issue. Or, to help a Cambodian patient to better regulate anger, one can use the Cambodian proverb, "If you don't become angry 1 time, it gains you 100 days of happiness." Also, to help a Cambodian patient to talk more openly about current issues of distress, one can use the proverb, "Don't *reek* by yourself," in which *reek* means "to carry a package at either end of a pole that is balanced at the shoulder." Or, among African American teenagers, the term "rebound" is a powerful motivator that is increasingly used as a reminder that you can recover after a missed "shot" or opportunity.

In the Spanish language, multiple tropes describe negative events in terms of images of suffocation or drowning.[36] To encourage a patient to talk about trauma memories, one may use the expression, "*desahogarse*," which literally means to "undrown yourself," and refers to talking about what is bothering you, with the connotation that not talking about such things is a kind of drowning.

Appropriate cultural analogies can also be used to create positive expectancy about treatment and to promote adherence. These can be used to promote positive expectancy. At the beginning of therapy, to promote adherence of a Cambodian patient to treatment and to create positive expectancy, we state that the treatment is like making a certain traditional noodle dish (*num beunycok*). Preparing that dish involves several steps that include making a paste, making noodles from the paste, and making the sauce. We explain that each part of the therapy, each lesson taught, is like a step in making this dish, and that one must wait until the end of therapy to know exactly what has been accomplished.

Presenting Cognitive Behavioral Therapy Information and Techniques in Terms of the Local Psychology, Physiology, and Spiritual Tradition

Every culture will have a certain set of ideas about how to manage negative affect and negative events, which range from ethnopsychology instantiated in proverb to formal religious practices and treatises. Those ideas may be incorporated to help teach CBT principles. Often these teachings involve metaphor and hence are related to the previous section. In the case of the Cambodian Buddhism, anger and other negative states are often compared to a fire. In fact, many traditional treatments involve a sort of cooling technology, such as anointing with waters that are considered supernaturally cooled. So then one can inform the patient that getting angry is like "bringing a fire into one's house," and one can give the analogy that, when angry, often there are 2 fires: the 1 fire is the anger caused by what the person did (eg, a child not listening to instructions) that is added to the fire of other similar events that are recalled to mind (eg, the child's father treating her badly).

Cultural Adaptation of Key Cognitive Behavioral Therapy Techniques

CBT techniques should be adapted for these groups to promote treatment tolerability, adherence, and overall efficacy (see previous discussion of addressing catastrophic cognitions). Exposure to trauma memory may need to be paired to emotion regulation to promote acceptability.[50] Visualizations may need to be modified. For example, in CA-CBT treatment, we have found it more efficacious to use imagery that promotes psychological flexibility and with certain Asian populations to do so by pairing the visualization of a wind-moved lotus to applied stretching. Or, in Latino populations, a study[51] found that relaxation imagery involving an allocentric (the idea that one defines self through social relationships) rather than an individualistic (the idea that one defines self through self attributes) orientation was more effective. In interoceptive exposure in CA-CBT, we do positive reassociations of somatic sensations to culturally appropriate images. Among Cambodian refugees, when doing head rolling, we have the patient imagine various traditional games: a game in which a person runs around in circles while holding a scarf (lea geunsaeng), or another game in which the person runs to get a stick that has been hit into the distance, all the while humming, making it impossible to inhale. Among Latinos, we have the patient imagine playing traditional games that induced considerable dizziness: playing the piñata game, which involves being blindfolded and spun around, or playing gallinita ciega. In these games, the person is spun until very dizzy. These are also examples of cultural grounding because locally salient practices and imagery are used.

Reducing Stigma

Stigma can be reduced by informing the patient that this anxiety and depressive disorder is treatable and that treatments, such as medication, will improve the condition. It is also extremely helpful in order to reduce stigma to frame the treatment in a way that it is not perceived as stigmatizing. For example, one can frame the treatment as reducing a somatic symptom, such as dizziness, or improving vegetative functions, such as sleep or appetite; these symptom conditions are not stigmatizing. The patient then may describe their treatment to others in their family or social network as targeting those non-stigmatizing treatment targets. Specific stigma-related beliefs should be addressed.

Culturally Indicated Transitional Rituals

If the culture has purification or transitional rites, such as steam bath rituals among Cambodian refugees, Vietnamese refugees, and certain American Indian groups,[52] the patient should be encouraged to perform that rite at the end of treatment. This creates a sense of closure and of positive transformation. These rituals also have healing properties in themselves. For example, the steaming ritual induces a somatic state that is analogous to an anxiety state: flushing and shortness of breath. It thus acts as exposure to those sensations and as a positive reimagining of them; the steaming ritual often involves fragrant substances and symbolic objects that become associated with, and conditioned to, the somatic sensations. This type of healing results in new positive semiotic networks for certain sensations; that is, creates new positive associations to sensations. These rituals also create a positive self-image (of being transformed in certain specific ways) and positive memories, and provide a positive world image, a cosmology. Also, positive expectancy is increased because the person has a sense of being positively transformed.

SUMMARY

This article has attempted to illustrate how CBT can be adapted to treat refugees and ethnic minorities with anxiety and depressive disorders. A model of the cultural influences on the development of anxiety and depressive disorders (see **Fig. 1**) and a model of explanatory model bridging (see **Fig. 2**) were presented. Key CA treatment components (see **Table 1**) that aim to address the processes in the model (see **Fig. 1**) were described and illustrated using examples, especially those from the first author's CA-CBT for trauma-related disorder. More generally, the cultural grounding of CBT with the goal of making it contextually sensitive CBT was outlined.

The approach in this article is consistent with recommendations about how to make treatment more culturally competent, a basic idea of which is that the efficacy of treatment increases as local meanings and sources of resilience[6,53–55] are considered: addressing locally emphasized somatic symptoms and syndromes; modifying catastrophic cognitions, including local metaphors and proverbs; comparing CBT techniques to local practices; and incorporating aspects of the local religious and healing traditions.[40] These are ways to culturally ground CBT in order to develop contextually sensitive CBT.

Future studies should examine, through mediational analyses and dismantling studies, whether the model of the cultural influences on the generation of anxiety and depressive disorders is accurate, and whether the interventions identified in the model lead to improvement. Future studies should explore how the recommendations advanced in this article are applicable to psychological disorders other than anxiety and depression.[56,57]

REFERENCES

1. Hofmann SG, Smits JA. Cognitive-behavioral therapy for adult anxiety disorders: a meta-analysis of randomized placebo-controlled trials. J Clin Psychiatry 2008; 69(4):621–32.

2. Bass JK, Annan J, McIvor Murray S, et al. Controlled trial of psychotherapy for Congolese survivors of sexual violence. N Engl J Med 2013;368(23):2182–91.

3. Drozdek B, Kamperman AM, Tol WA, et al. Seven-year follow-up study of symptoms in asylum seekers and refugees with PTSD treated with trauma-focused groups. J Clin Psychol 2014;70(4):376–87.

4. Hinton DE. Assessment and treatment in non-Western countries. In: Emmelkamp P, Ehring E, editors. The Wiley handbook of anxiety disorders. Hoboken (NJ): Wiley; 2014. p. 1268–78.

5. Hinton DE, Pich V, Hofmann SG, et al. Mindfulness and acceptance techniques as applied to refugee and ethnic minority populations: examples from culturally adapted CBT (CA-CBT). Cogn Behav Pract 2013;20:33–46.

6. Hwang WC, Myers HF, Chiu E, et al. Culturally adapted cognitive-behavioral therapy for Chinese Americans with depression: a randomized controlled trial. Psychiatr Serv 2015;66(10):1035–42.

7. Murray LK, Dorsey S, Haroz E, et al. A common elements approach for adult mental health problems in low- and middle-income countries. Cogn Behav Pract 2014;21:111–23.

8. Naeem F, Waheed W, Gobbi M, et al. Preliminary evaluation of culturally sensitive CBT for depression in Pakistan: findings from developing culturally-sensitive CBT project (DCCP). Behav Cogn Psychother 2011;39:165–73.

9. Nickerson A, Bryant RA, Silove D, et al. A critical review of psychological treatments of posttraumatic stress disorder in refugees. Clin Psychol Rev 2011; 31(3):399–417.

10. Crumlish N, O'Rourke K. A systematic review of treatments for post-traumatic stress disorder among refugees and asylum-seekers. J Nerv Ment Dis 2010; 198(4):237–51.

11. Griner D, Smith TB. Culturally adapted mental health intervention: a meta-analytic review. Psychotherapy 2006;43(4):531–48.

12. Benish SG, Quintana S, Wampold BE. Culturally adapted psychotherapy and the legitimacy of myth: a direct-comparison meta-analysis. J Couns Psychol 2011; 58(3):279–89.

13. Bernal G, Jiménez-Chafey MI, Domenech Rodríguez MD. Cultural adaptation of treatments: a resource for considering culture in evidence-based practic. Prof Psychol Res Pract 2009;40:361–8.

14. Hinton DE, Good BJ, editors. Culture and panic disorder. Palo Alto (CA): Stanford University Press; 2009.

15. Hinton DE, Good BJ, editors. Culture and PTSD: trauma in historical and global perspective. Pennsylvania: University of Pennsylvenia Press; 2016.

16. Kleinman A, Good BJ, editors. Culture and depression: studies in anthropology and cross-cultural psychiatry of affect and disorder. Berkeley (CA): University of California Press; 1985.

17. Hinton DE, Lewis-Fernández R, Kirmayer LJ, et al. Supplementary module 1: explanatory module. In: Lewis-Fernandez R, Aggarwal N, Hinton L, et al, editors. The DSM-5 handbook on the cultural formulation interview. Washington, DC: American Psychiatric Press; 2016. p. 53–67.

18. Hinton DE, Chhean D, Pich V, et al. A randomized controlled trial of cognitive-behavior therapy for Cambodian refugees with treatment-resistant PTSD and panic attacks: a cross-over design. J Trauma Stress 2005;18(6):617–29.

19. Hinton DE, Hofmann SG, Rivera E, et al. Culturally adapted CBT for Latino women with treatment-resistant PTSD: a pilot study comparing CA-CBT to applied muscle relaxation. Behav Res Ther 2011;49:275–80.

20. Hinton DE, Jalal B. Guidelines for the implementation of culturally sensitive CBT among refugees and in global contexts. Intervention 2014;12:78–93.

21. Hinton DE, Jalal B. Parameters for creating culturally sensitive CBT: implementing CBT in global settings. Cogn Behav Pract 2014;21:139–44.

22. Hinton DE, Pham T, Tran M, et al. CBT for Vietnamese refugees with treatment-resistant PTSD and panic attacks: a pilot study. J Trauma Stress 2004;17(5): 429–33.

23. Jalal B, Kruger Q, Hinton DH. Adaptation of CBT for a traumatized South African indigenous group (Sepedi): examples from culturally adapted somatic-focused CBT (CA-CBT). Cogntive and Behavioral Practice, in press.

24. Jalal B, Samir SW, Hinton DH. Adaptation of CBT for traumatized Egyptians: examples from culturally adapted CBT (CA-CBT). Cogntive and Behavioral Practice 2017;24:58–71.

25. Woodhead EL, Ivan II, Emery EE. An exploratory study of inducing positive expectancies for psychotherapy. Aging Ment Health 2012;16:162–6.

26. Lewis-Fernández R, Diaz N. The cultural formulation: a method for assessing cultural factors affecting the clinical encounter. Psychiatr Q 2002;73(4):271–95.

27. Sue DW, Sue D. Counseling the culturally diverse: theory and practice. Hoboken (NJ): Wiley; 2007.

28. Hinton DE, Hinton AL, Eng K-T, et al. PTSD and key somatic complaints and cultural syndromes among rural Cambodians: the results of a needs assessment survey. Med Anthropol Q 2012;29:147–54.

29. Hinton DE, Kredlow MA, Pich V, et al. The relationship of PTSD to key somatic complaints and cultural syndromes among Cambodian refugees attending a psychiatric clinic: the Cambodian Somatic Symptom and Syndrome Inventory (SSI). Transcult Psychiatr 2013;50:347–70.

30. Hinton DE, Hofmann SG, Pollack MH, et al. Mechanisms of efficacy of CBT for Cambodian refugees with PTSD: improvement in emotion regulation and orthostatic blood pressure response. CNS Neurosci Ther 2009;15(3):255–63.

31. Hinton DE, Reis R, de Jong J, et al. The "thinking a lot" idiom of distress and PTSD: an examination of their relationship among traumatized Cambodian refugees using the "thinking a lot" questionnaire. Med Anthropol Q 2015;29:357–80.

32. Hinton DE, Barlow DH, Reis R, et al. A transcultural model of the centrality of "thinking a lot" in psychopathologies across the globe and the process of localization: a Cambodian refugee example. Cult Med Psychiatry 2016;40(4):570–619.

33. Hinton DE, Pich V, Marques L, et al. Khyâl attacks: a key idiom of distress among traumatized Cambodian refugees. Cult Med Psychiatry 2010;34:244–78.

34. Hinton DE, Lewis-Fernández R. Idioms of distress among trauma survivors: subtypes and clinical utility. Cult Med Psychiatry 2010;34:209–18.

35. Hinton DE, Lewis-Fernández R. "Idioms of distress" (culturally salient indicators of distress) and anxiety disorders. In: Simpson HB, Neria Y, Lewis-Fernández R, et al, editors. Anxiety disorders: theory, research, and clinical perspectives. Cambridge (United Kingdom): Cambridge University Press; 2010. p. 127–38.

36. Hinton DE, Lewis-Fernández R, Pollack MH. A model of the generation of ataque de nervios: the role of fear of negative affect and fear of arousal symptoms. CNS Neurosci Ther 2009;15:264–75.

37. Hinton DE, Rasmussen A, Nou L, et al. Anger, PTSD, and the nuclear family: a study of Cambodian refugees. Soc Sci Med 2009;69:1387–94.

38. Hagengimana A, Hinton DE. Ihahamuka, a Rwandan syndrome of response to the genocide: blocked flow, spirit assault, and shortness of breath. In: Hinton DE, Good BJ, editors. Culture and panic disorder. Stanford (CA): Stanford University Press; 2009. p. 205–29.

39. Hinton DE, Hinton A, Chhean D, et al. Nightmares among Cambodian refugees: the breaching of concentric ontological security. Cult Med Psychiatry 2009;33: 219–65.

40. Hinton DE, Kredlow MA, Bui E, et al. Treatment change of somatic symptoms and cultural syndromes among Cambodian refugees with PTSD. Depress Anxiety 2012;29:148–55.

41. Hinton DE, Lewis-Fernández R. The cross-cultural validity of posttraumatic stress disorder: implications for DSM-5. Depress Anxiety 2011;28:783–801.
42. Hinton DE, Otto MW. Symptom presentation and symptom meaning among traumatized Cambodian refugees: relevance to a somatically focused cognitive-behavior therapy. Cogn Behav Pract 2006;13:249–60.
43. Carlson CR, Curran SL. Stretch-based relaxation training. Patient Educ Couns 1994;23(1):5–12.
44. Ghoncheh S, Smith JC. Progressive muscle relaxation, yoga stretching, and ABC relaxation theory. J Clin Psychol 2004;60(1):131–6.
45. Öst LG, Westling B. Applied relaxation vs. cognitive behavior therapy in the treatment of panic disorder. Behav Res Ther 1995;33:145–58.
46. Clark DM. A cognitive approach to panic. Behaviour Research and Therapy 1986;24:461–70.
47. Aviera A. "Dichos" therapy group: a therapeutic use of Spanish language proverbs with hospitalized Spanish-speaking psychiatric patients. Cult Divers Ment Health 1996;2:73–87.
48. Hyman R, Ortiz J, Añez L, et al. Culture and clinical practice recommendations for working with Puerto Ricans and other Latinos in the United States. Prof Psychol Res Pract 2006;37:694–701.
49. Otto MW. Stories and metaphors in therapy. Cogn Behav Pract 2000;7:166–72.
50. Hinton DE, Rivera E, Hofmann SG, et al. Adapting CBT for traumatized refugees and ethnic minority patients: examples from culturally adapted CBT (CA-CBT). Transcult Psychiatr 2012;49:340–65.
51. La Roche M, D'Angelo E, Gualdron L, et al. Culturally sensitive guided imagery for allocentric Latinos: a pilot study. Psychotherapy (Chic) 2006;43:555–60.
52. Silver SM, Wilson JP. Native American healing and purification rituals for war stress. In: Wilson JP, Harel Z, Kahana B, editors. Human adaptation to extreme stress: from the Holocaust to Vietnam. New York: Plenum; 1988. p. 337–56.
53. Healey P, Stager ML, Woodmass K, et al. Cultural adaptations to augment health and mental health services: a systematic review. BMC Health Serv Res 2017; 17(1):8.
54. La Roche M, Lustig K. Cultural adaptations: unpacking the meaning of culture. Scientific Rev Ment Health Pract 2010;7:26–30.
55. Sue D, Ivey A, Pedersen P. Theories of multicultural counseling and therapy. Mason (OH): Cengage Learning Press; 2007.
56. Foa EB, Rothbaum BO. Treating the trauma of rape: cognitive-behavioral therapy for PTSD. New York: Guilford; 1998.
57. Resick P, Schnicke M. Cognitive processing therapy for rape victims. London: Sage Publications; 1996.

Can Cognitive Behavioral Therapy for Anxiety and Depression Be Improved with Pharmacotherapy? A Meta-analysis

David F. Tolin, PhD

KEYWORDS

- Cognitive-behavioral therapy • Drug treatment • Antidepressants
- Anxiety disorders • Depression

KEY POINTS

- Antidepressant and anxiolytic medications do not consistently or markedly enhance the effects of CBT for patients with anxiety or depressive disorders.
- Antidepressant medications may be efficacious second-line treatments for patients failing to respond to CBT.
- Novel agents that are thought to potentiate the neurobiological mechanisms of CBT are promising but await further study.

ROOM FOR IMPROVEMENT IN COGNITIVE-BEHAVIORAL THERAPY

The efficacy of cognitive-behavioral therapy (CBT) is well established in the treatment of anxiety and depressive disorders. Meta-analyses of controlled trials indicates a moderate-sized superiority for CBT versus placebo (PBO) treatment,[1,2] and small to moderate-sized superiority over alternative psychological treatments such as psychodynamic therapy.[3] However, there is clearly room for improvement: across trials, as many as half of patients receiving CBT are considered nonresponders at posttreatment.[4–7]

THE POTENTIAL FOR PHARMACOLOGIC AUGMENTATION

Thus, an important question is whether pharmacologic treatment, added to CBT, can improve outcomes over CBT alone. The efficacy of medications as monotherapies for

Disclosures: Dr D.F. Tolin has received recent research funding from Palo Alto Health Sciences, Inc. and Pfizer. He receives royalties from Guilford Press, Oxford University Press, Turner Publishing, and Springer.
The Institute of Living, Anxiety Disorders Center, 200 Retreat Avenue, Hartford, CT 06106, USA
E-mail address: david.tolin@hhchealth.org

Psychiatr Clin N Am 40 (2017) 715–738
http://dx.doi.org/10.1016/j.psc.2017.08.007
0193-953X/17/© 2017 Elsevier Inc. All rights reserved.

anxiety and depressive disorders is reasonably well established, although significant concerns about reporting standards (some of which could apply to CBT trials as well as pharmacotherapy trials) have been raised.[8,9] Across studies, antidepressant medications, including selective serotonin reuptake inhibitors (SSRIs), serotonin-norepinephrine reuptake inhibitors (SNRIs), tricyclic antidepressants, and monoamine oxidase inhibitors (MAOIs) show superiority over PBO for depression,[10–12] although the overall effect is small,[13] and may be clinically meaningful only in more severe cases.[14,15] Among the anxiety disorders, the antidepressant medications, as well as anxiolytic medications including benzodiazepines and azapirones, also show a superiority to PBO across studies, with medium effects overall.[16] When medications and CBT have been compared directly, across studies the effects are roughly equivalent, at least in the short term.[2,16–21]

THE NEED TO EXAMINE PLACEBO-CONTROLLED TRIALS OF PSYCHOPHARMACOLOGIC AUGMENTATION

Previous systematic reviews have examined whether the combination of these treatments is better than CBT alone. These reviews have generally shown a small advantage of combined treatment over CBT alone, although there may be an increased risk of relapse when medications are withdrawn.[22–27] Importantly, however, an examination of CBT + medications versus CBT alone cannot facilitate an adequate understanding of the incremental efficacy of medications. In the absence of a PBO control condition, there is no way to determine the effects of the medication, either positive or negative. The PBO response rate in anxiety disorders is substantial[28]; in one systematic review, pill PBO was demonstrated to increase the probability of response in panic disorder with agoraphobia (PD/A) by 26%.[29]

However, the PBO effect also may have the reverse effect in some cases: when patients with PD/A treated with alprazolam (ALP) versus PBO plus CBT rated the extent to which they believed that their treatment gains were attributable to medication or to their own efforts, those who attributed their gains to medication exhibited a greater loss of gains following discontinuation than did those who had attributed their gains to their own efforts during treatment.[30] Additionally, when patients with specific phobia (SpP) treated with exposure plus pill PBO were told that the pill had anxiolytic properties that would make exposure easier, they were more likely to relapse (39%) after treatment than were patients who were told that the pill had stimulating properties that would make exposure more difficult (0%), or those who were told that the pill had no effect on exposure (0%).[31] Thus, there may be both PBO and "nocebo"[32] effects of adding medications to CBT, beyond the specific pharmacologic effects of the medication itself. The aim of the present review was to examine the efficacy of pharmacologic augmentation of CBT by synthesizing studies that randomized patients to CBT + medications versus CBT + PBO.

The present review considers 3 distinct methods of pharmacologic augmentation of CBT. *First*, studies in which CBT was applied concurrently with a medication also used as a monotherapy (eg, CBT plus an SSRI) were examined. *Second*, studies in which pharmacologic treatment was administered following CBT nonresponse, rather than concurrent administration for all patients, were examined. This strategy relates to the practice of stepped care,[33,34] in which treatments are added sequentially only after nonresponse to the initial trial. *Third*, the analysis examines studies that used novel agents, not prescribed as monotherapies, to augment CBT. These studies were limited to the anxiety disorders, in which there has been increasing interest in compounds that do not treat the anxiety directly, but rather are thought to potentiate the mechanisms by which CBT (specifically exposure therapy) exerts its effects.[35] Two compounds that potentiate activity in the N-methyl-D-aspartic acid (NMDA) receptor in basolateral amygdala (implicated in fear extinction[36]) include D-cycloserine (DCS), which enhances fear extinction in animals,[37] and Org 25,935 (ORG), a glycine uptake inhibitor that enhances working memory in animals.[38] Three other compounds proposed to augment exposure therapy increase activity in the medial prefrontal cortex (mPFC), thought to be critical to the extinction of learned fear[39–41]: yohimbine (YOH), an α2-adrenergic receptor antagonist that enhances fear extinction in animals[42,43]; methylene blue (MB), an autoxidizing agent that enhances fear extinction in animals[44,45]; and oxytocin (OXT), a neuropeptide that disrupts signals from the amygdala to the autonomic nervous system[46,47] enhances (normalizes) resting state functional connectivity.

METHOD
Data Selection

A search was conducted on PsycINFO (1967–January 2017) using the terms (Cognitive Therapy or Cognitive Behavior Therapy or CBT or Behavior Therapy or Exposure Therapy) and (Anxiety Disorders or Phobia or Posttraumatic Stress Disorder or Obsessive Compulsive Disorder or Panic Disorder or Generalized Anxiety Disorder or Social Anxiety or Major Depressive Disorder or Major Depression or Dysthymic Disorder or Persistent Depressive Disorder) and (Medication or Drug Therapy or Antidepressant or Benzodiazepines or Augmentation), limited to peer-reviewed journals published in English and listed as clinical trials, empirical studies, longitudinal studies, prospective studies, or treatment outcome studies. Recent empirical and review articles were also searched for additional references. Criteria for inclusion were as follows:

1. Double-blind randomized controlled trials (RCTs) that included a CBT + medication condition and a CBT + PBO condition (other arms, when included, were not analyzed here). Studies of adults or children were accepted. Medication lead-in or extension periods were allowed, so long as there was a simultaneous application of CBT + medications.
2. Clearly defined CBT protocol (Internet-based and self-directed CBT were also included, but eclectic psychotherapies were not).
3. Participants had a clear primary *Diagnostic and Statistical Manual of Mental Disorders* (DSM) diagnosis of an anxiety disorder (categorized according to DSM-IV[48]) or unipolar depressive disorder (anxiety and depression within severe medical conditions, comorbid with substance use or developmental disorders, remitted illnesses, or treatments aimed at symptoms other than anxiety and depression were not included; student samples were also not included unless they met DSM criteria for an anxiety or depressive disorder).
4. Used standardized (reliable and valid) self-report or interview-based measures of the symptoms of the disorder being treated (global measures, functional outcomes, behavioral avoidance tests, and biomarker outcomes were not analyzed). When more than one such measure was included, effect sizes were aggregated across outcome measures. Responder rates were included only when they were based on a cutoff on a standardized measure of the symptoms of the disorder.
5. Study was judged to be a clinical trial rather than a preclinical study of mechanisms of action.
6. Provided data (eg, means and SDs, or proportions of responders when such data were not available) or statistics (eg, change scores or *F* values) that could be used to calculate an effect size. Posttreatment was defined as the last assessment

collected during (or immediately following) active treatment. Follow-up was defined as the last assessment (up to 3 years) after treatment had been discontinued (in some cases, the last follow-up analysis was published in a separate article).

As shown in **Fig. 1**, 1194 articles were considered for inclusion. Of these, 1126 were excluded (a list of excluded articles is available from the author); the most common reasons were absence of an RCT design, or lack of either a CBT + medication or CBT + PBO group. This process resulted in 68 studies that met inclusion criteria.

Data Analytic Strategy

Random-effects model meta-analytic strategies[49] were used with Comprehensive Meta-Analysis.[50] When possible, effect size estimates were calculated from the mean and SD of measures at pretreatment and posttreatment (and at follow-up, where applicable). When these data were not provided in the published article, effect sizes were estimated from interaction F values, mean and SD change scores, or mean change scores with t or P values within groups. Categorical outcomes (eg, response rates) were included only when continuous data were not available.

For each comparison of CBT + medication versus CBT + PBO, the Hedges g (weighted by inverse variance) was calculated. Hedges g is a small-sample correction of Cohen's d, for which values of 0.2, 0.5, and 0.8 are conventionally accepted to represent small, medium, and large effects, respectively.[51] Calculation of g for pre-post designs requires an estimate of the correlation (r) between the pretreatment

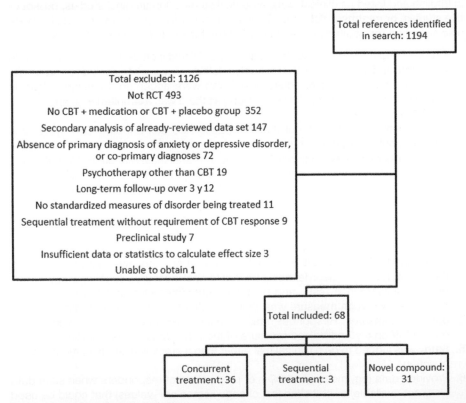

Fig. 1. Flowchart of study inclusion.

and posttreatment scores; because this was not available in published reports, r was conservatively estimated at 0.7 according to the recommendation of Rosenthal.[52] For ease of interpretation, pooled g estimates were also converted to number needed to treat (NNT) using the formula provided by Furukawa,[53,54] using an estimated overall 50% response rate in CBT + PBO.[4–7] NNT, in this case, refers to the number of patients who would have to receive CBT with medication to obtain 1 more favorable outcome over CBT with PBO. The I^2 statistic was used to assess the percentage of variation due to true heterogeneity rather than chance and is interpreted as follows: 25% = little heterogeneity, 50% = moderate heterogeneity, and 75% = high heterogeneity.[55] Significance of heterogeneity was established using the Q statistic.

From the literature search described previously, 36 articles were included in the concurrent treatment analysis (**Table 1**) that represented posttreatment and/or follow-up analyses of double-blind, RCTs of concurrent CBT + medications versus CBT + PBO (other arms, when used, are not reviewed here). Concurrent medications were divided into antidepressant and anxiolytic groups. For each class, the effect of medications was compared across diagnoses and across drug class. Only 3 double-blind RCTs of concurrent CBT + medications versus CBT + PBO for patients failing to respond adequately to CBT monotherapy were identified and included (**Table 2**). Thirty-one articles (**Table 3**) were included in the novel agent analysis representing double-blind, RCTs of concurrent CBT + novel agents versus CBT + PBO (other arms, when used, are not reviewed here).

RESULTS
Concurrent Cognitive-Behavior Therapy with Antidepressant Medication

As shown in **Table 4**, the pooled effect size for antidepressants was small at posttreatment, with an NNT of 7.7. At follow-up (after medication discontinuation), the pooled effect size was negative and in the negligible range. Thus, the addition of antidepressants confers a small advantage over CBT monotherapy at posttreatment, although this advantage is lost when medications are discontinued.

Antidepressant Medication by Diagnosis

There was no significant between-group heterogeneity according to diagnosis at posttreatment ($Q = 6.32$, $P = .18$) or at follow-up ($Q = 3.65$, $P = .30$). Thus, the additive effect of antidepressant medications does not appear to be significantly stronger for any specific anxiety or depressive disorder (although a range is noted, from $g = 0.17$ for social phobia [SoP] to $g = 0.63$ for posttraumatic stress disorder [PTSD]). For anxiety disorders, the additive effect of antidepressants over PBO was small, with an NNT of 9.1 at posttreatment, and negative and negligible at follow-up. Similarly, for depressive disorders, the effect was small, with an NNT of 7.5 at posttreatment, and negative and negligible at follow-up. Thus, the small benefit of additive antidepressant medications that is eliminated on medication discontinuation is seen across the anxiety and depressive disorders. Significant within-group heterogeneity was found only for PD/A at posttreatment; visual inspection of **Table 1** suggests that this was driven by a single study showing a treatment-attenuating effect of the MAOI moclobemide.

Antidepressant medication by drug class

There was significant between-group heterogeneity according to medication at posttreatment ($Q = 32.05$, $P = .001$), although no significant between-group heterogeneity was found at follow-up ($Q = 9.20$, $P = .10$). At posttreatment, tricyclics were associated with a medium effect, with an NNT of 5.2. SSRIs/SNRIs were associated with a

Table 1
Randomized trials of concurrent CBT with medication versus concurrent CBT with pill placebo

Study Name	Medication	Diagnosis	Posttreatment g	95% CI	Follow-up g	95% CI
Appleby et al,[78] 1997[a]	FLU	DEP	0.35	−0.01–0.70	—	—
Barlow et al,[79] 2000[b]	IMI	PD/A	0.71	0.35–1.06	−0.23	−0.57–0.12
Bellack et al,[80] 1981	AMI	DEP	0.04	−0.42–0.51	—	—
Beutler et al,[81] 1987	ALP	DEP	−1.06	−1.67 to −0.45	−0.14	−0.66–0.38
Blomhoff et al,[82] 2001; Haug et al,[83] 2003	SER	SoP	0.16	0.35–1.06	−0.34	−0.65 to −0.03
Bond et al,[84] 2002	BUS	GAD	0.71	−0.10–1.53	—	—
Chaudhry et al,[85] 1998	AMN	DEP	0.73	0.30–1.16	—	—
Clark et al,[86] 2003	FLU	SoP	0.28	−0.33–0.89	—	—
Cohen et al,[87] 2007	SER	PTSD	0.28	−0.18–0.75	—	—
Cottraux et al,[88] 1990; Cottraux et al,[89] 1993	FLV	OCD	0.42	−0.27–1.12	0.38	−0.32–1.10
Cottraux et al,[90] 1995	BUS	PD/A	0.38	−0.10–1.53	0.44	0.10–0.77
Davidson et al,[91] 2004	FLU	SoP	−0.02	−0.28–0.23	—	—
de Beurs et al,[92] 1995; de Beurs et al,[93] 1999	FLV	PD/A	1.50	0.85–2.16	0.28	−0.36–0.93
Echeburua et al,[94] 1993	ALP	PD/A	−0.11	−1.04–0.82	—	—
Fahy et al,[95] 1992	CMI	PD/A	1.10	0.45–1.74	—	—
Fahy et al,[95] 1992	LOF	PD/A	0.47	−0.14–1.08	—	—
Gingnell et al,[96] 2016	ESC	SoP	0.43	0.10–1.08	—	—
Hohagen et al,[97] 1998	FLV	OCD	0.53	−0.03–1.09	—	—
Loerch et al,[98] 1999	MOC	PD/A	−0.61	−1.35–0.13	−0.44	−0.88–0.00
Marks et al,[99] 1983	IMI	PD/A	0.54	−0.05–1.12	0.18	−0.40–0.77
Murphy et al,[100] 1984; Simons et al,[101] 1986	NOR	DEP	0.26	−0.29–0.82	0.36	−0.47–1.18
Peter et al,[102] 2000	FLV	OCD	0.78	0.09–1.48	—	—
Power et al,[103] 1990	DIA	GAD	1.02	0.36–1.68	—	—
Ravindran et al,[104] 1999	SER	DEP	0.87	0.39–1.77	—	—
Roth et al,[105] 1987	IMI	PD/A	0.74	0.39–1.77	—	—
Rothbaum et al,[106] 2014	ALP	PTSD	−0.06	−0.33–0.21	−0.18	−0.46–0.09
Schneier et al,[107] 2012	PAR	PTSD	1.06	0.38–1.73	—	—
Sharp et al,[108] 1996	FLV	PD/A	0.16	−0.36–0.68	—	—
Stein et al,[109] 2000	PAR	PD/A	0.20	−0.29–0.68	—	—
Storch et al,[110] 2013	SER	OCD	0.07	−0.21–0.35	—	—
Telch et al,[111] 1985	IMI	PD/A	1.47	0.77–2.18	—	—
Wardle et al,[112] 1994	DIA	PD/A	−0.63	−1.13 to −0.12	—	—
Wilson,[113] 1982	AMI	DEP	−0.16	−0.76–0.44	−0.43	−1.03–0.18

$P<.05$.

Abbreviations: ALP, alprazolam; AMI, amitriptyline; AMN, amineptine; BUS, buspirone; CBT, cognitive-behavioral therapy; CI, confidence interval; CMI, clomipramine; DEP, depression; DIA, diazepam; ESC, escitalopram; FLU, fluoxetine; FLV, fluvoxamine; GAD, generalized anxiety disorder; IMI, imipramine; LOF, lofepramine; MOC, moclobemide; NOR, nortriptyline; OCD, obsessive-compulsive disorder; PAR, paroxetine; PD/A, panic disorder (and/or agoraphobia); PTSD, posttraumatic stress disorder; SER, sertraline; SoP, social phobia; —, no data.

[a] The 6-session CBT was included.
[b] The postmaintenance interview was included.

Table 2 Randomized trials of sequential administration of medications versus placebo with CBT								
Study Name	Medication	Diagnosis	g	95% CI	Q	I^2	NNT
Simon et al,[114] 2008	PAR	PTSD	−0.36	−1.17–0.46	—	—	—
Kampman et al,[115] 2002	PAR	PD/A	0.81	0.16–1.46	—	—	3.4
Stewart et al,[116] 1993	IMI	DEP	2.04	0.70–3.38	—	—	2.1
Overall			0.57	0.10–1.04	10.14[a]	80.28	4.6

Abbreviations: CBT, cognitive-behavioral therapy; CI, confidence interval; DEP, depression; IMI, imipramine; NNT, number needed to treat; PAR, paroxetine; PD/A, panic disorder (and/or agoraphobia); PTSD, posttraumatic stress disorder.
[a] P <.05.

small effect, with an NNT of 9.1. The one study of an MAOI was associated with a negative effect. Thus, the available evidence suggests that tricyclics are associated with the greatest augmentation effect. Significant within-group heterogeneity was seen at posttreatment in the SSRIs paroxetine (PAR) and sertraline (SER); **Table 1** shows a discrepancy between the 2 studies of PAR, whereas only 1 of the 3 SER studies showed a large effect.

Anxiolytic medication by diagnosis
One study used ALP in the treatment of depression in older adults; that study was associated with a large negative effect for the additional medication. Although benzodiazepines are not uncommon in the treatment of older adults with depression,[56–58] most experts do not currently recommend this treatment.[59–61] Because this study represents both a contested prescribing practice and a statistical outlier, **Table 5** presents the results with and without that study. Only the analyses excluding that study are discussed here. Overall, the additive effect of anxiolytics over PBO was negligible, with an NNT of 18.0 at posttreatment and 35.8 at follow-up. However, significant between-group heterogeneity was found across diagnoses at posttreatment ($Q = 10.98, P = .004$), with a large effect in generalized anxiety disorder (GAD) versus negligible and negative effects in PD/A and PTSD. Significant between-group heterogeneity also was found across diagnoses at follow-up ($Q = 7.91, P = .005$), with a small to medium effect in PD/A versus a negative and negligible effect for PTSD. Thus, the available evidence suggests that concurrent anxiolytic medications confer a stronger benefit for GAD than for other disorders at posttreatment; 1 study also suggests a potentially enduring effect in PD/A after medication discontinuation. Significant within-group heterogeneity was found at posttreatment only for PD/A; visual inspection of **Table 1** suggests that this was due to a treatment-attenuating effect of benzodiazepines versus a small positive effect in one study of buspirone (BUS) for PD/A.

Anxiolytic medication by drug class
Marginal ($Q = 5.65, P = .06$) between-group heterogeneity was found across the anxiolytic medications at posttreatment, with benzodiazepines associated with a negligible and negative effect, and BUS associated with a small to medium effect and an NNT of 6.1. At follow-up, significant between-group heterogeneity was also across medications ($Q = 7.91, P = .005$), with a negative and negligible effect for ALP and a small to medium effect for BUS, with an NNT of 5.9. Significant within-group heterogeneity was seen for diazepam (DIA); **Table 1** shows a large positive effect in one study of GAD and a medium negative effect in another study of PD/A.

Table 3
Randomized trials of concurrent CBT with novel agents versus concurrent CBT with pill placebo

Study Name	Medication	Diagnosis	Posttreatment g	95% CI	Follow-up g	95% CI
Acheson et al,[117] 2015	OXT	SpP	−0.78	−1.36 to −0.19	—	—
Andersson et al,[118] 2015	DCS	OCD	0.33	−0.02–0.67	0.12	−0.23–0.46
de Kleine et al,[119] 2012	DCS	PTSD	1.80	1.40–2.20	0.27	−0.06–0.61
Difede et al,[120] 2014	DCS	PTSD	0.83	0.03–1.62	1.42	0.57–2.28
Farrell et al,[121] 2013	DCS	OCD	0.21	−0.69–1.12	0.72	−0.22–1.66
Guastella et al,[122] 2008	DCS	SoP	0.60	0.29–0.90	0.49	0.18–0.79
Guastella et al,[123] 2009	OXT	SoP	−0.31	−0.75–0.13	−0.41	−0.94–0.13
Hofmann et al,[124] 2006	DCS	SoP	0.57	0.04–1.10	0.84	0.25–1.43
Hofmann et al,[125] 2013	DCS	SoP	0.25	0.04–0.46	−0.12	−0.33–0.10
Kushner et al,[126] 2007	DCS	OCD	−0.18	−0.86–0.50	−0.41	−1.09–0.28
Litz et al,[127] 2012	DCS	PTSD	−0.93	−1.48 to −0.37	−0.37	−0.91–0.16
Mataix-Cols et al,[128] 2014	DCS	OCD	0.23	−0.50–0.97	0.08	−0.66–0.81
Meyerbroeker et al,[129] 2012	YOH	SpP	0.21	−0.20–0.62	—	—
Nations et al,[38] 2012	ORG	PD/A	0.25	−0.14–0.65	0.73	0.33–1.14
Nave et al,[130] 2012	DCS	SpP	0.42	−0.43–1.26	—	—
Otto et al,[131] 2010	DCS	PD/A	1.08	0.31–1.86	0.79	0.04–1.54
Otto et al,[132] 2016	DCS	PD/A	0.32	0.03–0.62	—	—
Powers et al,[133] 2009	YOH	SpP	0.17	−0.39–0.72	1.40	0.78–2.02
Ressler et al,[134] 2004	DCS	SpP	1.02	0.45–1.59	—	—
Rapee et al,[135] 2016	DCS	Mix	0.09	−0.29–0.47	—	—
Rothbaum et al,[106] 2014	DCS	PTSD	−0.10	−0.37–0.16	0.06	−0.21–0.32
Scheeringa and Weems,[136] 2014	DCS	PTSD	−0.06	−0.57–0.46	−0.09	−0.60–0.42
Siegmund et al,[73] 2011	DCS	PD/A	0.23	−0.39–0.84	—	—
Smits et al,[137] 2014	YOH	SoP	0.81	0.18–1.44	—	—
Storch et al,[138] 2007	DCS	OCD	−0.32	−0.87–0.23	−0.89	−1.15 to −0.03
Storch et al,[139] 2010	DCS	OCD	0.49	−0.22–1.20	—	—
Storch et al,[140] 2016	DCS	OCD	0.13	−0.20–0.46	—	—
Tart et al,[141] 2013	DCS	SpP	0.00	−0.50–0.50	−0.15	−0.65–0.36
Telch et al,[142] 2014	MB	SpP	—	—	0.36	−0.24–0.96
Wilhelm et al,[143] 2008	DCS	OCD	1.06	0.21–1.91	1.09	0.23–1.92
Zoellner et al,[144] 2017	MB	PTSD	−0.01	−0.49–0.48	0.71	0.20–1.20

Abbreviations: CBT, cognitive-behavioral therapy; CI, confidence interval; DCS, D-cycloserine; MB, methylene blue; OCD, obsessive-compulsive disorder; ORG, Org 25,935; OXT, oxytocin; PD/A, panic disorder (and/or agoraphobia); PTSD, posttraumatic stress disorder; SoP, social phobia; SpP, specific phobia; YOH, yohimbine; —, no data.

Cognitive-Behavioral Therapy with Medication for Patients Nonresponsive to Cognitive-Behavioral Therapy Monotherapy

As shown in **Table 2**, the 3 controlled trials of medications versus PBO for CBT non-responders showed a medium to large advantage overall for medications, although

Table 4

Summaries of trials of concurrent CBT with antidepressant medications versus concurrent CBT with pill placebo, by diagnosis and by medication

Diagnosis	Posttreatment						Follow-up					
	k	g	95% CI	Q	I^2	NNT	k	g	95% CI	Q	I^2	NNT
SoP	4	0.17	0.01–0.34	4.81	37.64	14.8	1	−0.34	−0.65 to −0.03	0.00	0.00	—
OCD	4	0.36	0.02–0.69	5.08	41.00	7.1	1	0.38	−0.32–1.07	0.00	0.00	6.8
PTSD	2	0.63	−0.12–1.39	3.42	70.79	4.2	0	—	—	—	—	—
PD/A	10	0.61	0.26–0.97	32.02[a]	71.89	4.4	4	−0.12	−0.42–0.18	4.85	38.17	—
Total anxiety	20	0.28	0.09–0.41	45.34[a]	—	9.1	6	−0.17	−0.38–0.03	4.85	—	—
DEP	6	0.34	0.06–0.62	9.96	49.78	7.5	2	−0.08	−0.82–0.65	2.24	55.41	—
Total depression	6	0.34	0.06–0.62	9.96	—	7.5	2	−0.08	−0.82–0.65	2.24	—	—

Medication	Posttreatment						Follow-up					
	k	g	95% CI	Q	I²	NNT	k	g	95% CI	Q	I²	NNT
AMI	2	−0.03	−0.39–0.32	0.28	0.00	—	1	−0.41	−0.99–0.17	0.00	0.00	—
NOR	1	0.26	−0.29–0.81	0.00	0.00	9.7	1	0.35	−0.46–1.15	0.00	0.00	7.3
LOF	1	0.47	−0.14–1.08	0.00	0.00	5.5	0	—	—	—	—	—
AMN	1	0.72	0.29–1.15	0.00	0.00	3.8	0	—	—	—	—	—
IMI	4	0.81	0.45–1.18	4.57	34.33	3.4	2	−0.09	−0.47–0.29	1.42	29.43	—
CMI	1	1.10	0.45–1.74	0.00	0.00	2.7	0	—	—	—	—	—
Total tricyclic	10	0.50	0.31–0.68	4.85	—	5.2	4	−0.11	−0.41–0.18	1.42	—	—
FLU	3	0.15	−0.11–0.41	3.07	34.97	16.8	0	—	—	—	—	—
SER	4	0.20	0.01–0.40	4.88	38.45	12.6	1	−0.34	−0.65–0.03	0.00	0.00	—
ESC	1	0.43	0.10–0.76	0.00	0.00	6.0	0	—	—	—	—	—
PAR	2	0.59	−0.25–1.44	4.12[a]	75.74	4.5	0	—	—	—	—	—
FLV	5	0.66	0.21–1.11	10.79[a]	62.94	4.1	2	0.32	−0.17–0.79	0.04	0.00	8.0
Total SSRI/SNRI	15	0.28	0.14–0.41	22.86[a]	—	9.1	3	−0.14	−0.39–0.12	0.04	—	—
MOC	1	−0.61	−1.35–0.13	0.00	0.00	—	1	−0.43	−0.86–0.00	0.00	0.00	—
Total MAOI	1	−0.61	−1.35–0.13	0.00	—	—	1	−0.44	−0.88–0.00	0.00	0.00	—
Total antidepressant	26	0.33	0.22–0.44	28.09[a]	—	7.7	8	−0.18	−0.35–0.00	1.46	—	—

Abbreviations: AMI, amitriptyline; AMN, amineptine; CBT, cognitive-behavioral therapy; CI, confidence interval; CMI, clomipramine; DEP, depression; ESC, escitalopram; FLU, fluvoxamine; FLV, fluoxetine; IMI, imipramine; MAOI, monoamine oxidase inhibitor; MOC, moclobemide; NNT, number needed to treat; NOR, nortriptyline; OCD, obsessive-compulsive disorder; PAR, paroxetine; PD/A, panic disorder (and/or agoraphobia); PTSD, post-traumatic stress disorder; SER, sertraline; SoP, social phobia; SSRI/SNRI, selective serotonin reuptake inhibitor/serotonin-norepinephrine reuptake inhibitor; —, no data.

[a] $P < .05$.

Table 5
Summaries of trials of concurrent CBT with anxiolytic medications versus concurrent CBT with pill placebo, by diagnosis and by medication

Diagnosis	Posttreatment						Follow-up					
	k	g	95% CI	Q	I²	NNT	k	g	95% CI	Q	I²	NNT
PTSD	1	−0.06	−0.33–0.21	0.00	0.00	—	1	−0.18	−0.45–0.09	0.00	0.00	—
PD/A	3	−0.10	−0.83–0.62	10.79[b]	81.47	—	1	0.43	0.10–0.76	0.00	0.00	6.0
GAD	2	0.90	0.39–1.41	0.33	0.00	3.2	—	—	—	—	—	—
Total Anxiety	6	0.13	−0.10–0.35	11.12[b]	—	19.3	2	0.07	−0.14–0.28	0.00	—	35.8
DEP	1	−1.03	−1.62 to −0.44	0.00	0.00	—	1	−0.14	−0.64–0.36	0.00	0.00	—
Total depression	1	−1.03	−1.62 to −0.44	0.00	—	—	1	−0.14	−0.66–0.38	0.00	0.00	—

Medication	Posttreatment						Follow-up					
	k	g	95% CI	Q	I²	NNT	k	g	95% CI	Q	I²	NNT
ALP	3	−0.40	−1.11–0.28	8.64[b]	76.85	—	2	−0.17	−0.41–0.07	0.02	0.00	—
ALP[a]	2	−0.06	−0.32–0.20	0.01	0.00	—	1	−0.18	−0.45–0.09	0.00	0.00	—
DIA	2	0.18	−1.43–1.80	15.22[b]	93.43	14.0	—	—	—	—	—	—
Total benzodiazepine	5	−0.31	−0.94–0.31	23.86[b]	—	—	2	−0.17	−0.41–0.07	0.02	—	—
Total benzodiazepine[a]	4	−0.06	−0.32–0.20	15.23[b]	—	—	1	−0.18	−0.45–0.09	0.00	—	—
BUS	2	0.42	0.12–0.73	0.57	0.00	6.1	1	0.44	0.10–0.77	0.00	0.00	5.9
Total azapirone	2	0.42	0.12–0.73	0.57	—	6.1	1	0.44	0.10–0.77	0.00	—	6.0
Total anxiolytic	7	0.28	0.01–0.56	24.42[b]	—	9.1	3	0.04	−0.16–0.23	0.02	—	62.7
Total anxiolytic[a]	6	0.14	−0.06–0.34	15.80[b]	—	18.0	2	0.07	−0.14–0.28	0.00	—	35.8

Abbreviations: ALP, alprazolam; BUS, buspirone; CBT, cognitive-behavioral therapy; CI, confidence interval; DEP, depression; DIA, diazepam; k, number of studies; NNT, number needed to treat; PD/A, panic disorder (and/or agoraphobia); PTSD, posttraumatic stress disorder; —, no data.
[a] Excluding the Beutler et al. (1987)[81] study.
[b] $P < .05$.

Table 6

Summaries of trials of concurrent CBT with novel agents versus concurrent CBT with pill placebo, by diagnosis and by medication

Diagnosis	Posttreatment						Follow-up					
	k	g	95% CI	Q	I²	NNT	k	g	95% CI	Q	I²	NNT
Mixed	1	0.09	−0.29−0.47	0.00	0.00	27.9	—	—	—	—	—	—
SpP	6	0.16	−0.28−0.61	19.46[a]	74.31	15.7	3	0.52	−0.37−1.42	14.70[a]	86.40	5.0
OCD	8	0.19	−0.04−0.43	9.87	29.10	13.3	6	0.10	−0.35−0.54	14.51[a]	65.54	25.1
PTSD	6	0.25	−0.52−1.02	85.96[a]	94.18	10.1	6	0.25	−0.10−0.61	18.67[a]	73.22	10.1
PD/A	4	0.36	0.11−0.62	3.86	22.23	7.1	3	0.43	−0.23−1.09	13.27[a]	84.92	6.0
SoP	6	0.41	0.10−0.71	16.22[a]	69.18	6.3	4	0.18	−0.29−0.66	19.61[a]	84.70	14.0
Overall	31	0.26	0.1−0.40	135.38[a]	—	9.7	22	0.24	0.02−0.45	80.76[a]	—	10.5

Medication	Posttreatment						Follow-up					
	k	g	95% CI	Q	I²	NNT	k	g	95% CI	Q	I²	NNT
OXT	2	−0.50	−0.96 to −0.05	1.58	36.87	—	1	−0.41	−0.94−0.13	0.00	0.00	—
MB	1	−0.01	−0.49−0.48	0.00	0.00	—	2	0.56	0.18−0.94	0.76	0.00	4.7
ORG	1	0.25	−0.14−0.65	0.00	0.00	10.1	1	0.73	0.33−1.14	0.00	0.00	3.7
DCS	24	0.35	0.14−0.56	114.72[a]	80.12	7.3	17	0.16	−0.04−0.35	50.92[a]	68.58	15.7
YOH	3	0.35	−0.01−0.70	2.84	29.63	7.3	1	1.40	0.78−2.02	0.00	0.00	2.4
Overall	31	0.26	0.1−0.40	135.38[a]	—	9.7	22	0.32	0.18−0.47	51.68[a]	—	8.0

DCS Trials Only	Posttreatment						Follow-up					
	k	g	95% CI	Q	I^2	NNT	k	g	95% CI	Q	I^2	NNT
Mixed	1	0.09	−0.29–0.47	0.00	0.00	27.9	—	—	—	—	—	—
OCD	8	0.19	−0.04–0.43	9.87	29.10	13.3	6	0.10	−0.35–0.54	14.51[a]	65.54	25.1
PTSD	5	0.31	−0.63–1.24	84.86[a]	95.29	8.2	5	0.16	−0.21–0.53	13.88[a]	71.18	15.7
PD/A	3	0.45	0.04–0.86	3.54	43.54	5.8	2	0.27	−0.59–1.14	4.75[a]	78.96	9.4
SpP	3	0.47	−0.20–1.14	6.91[a]	71.04	5.5	1	−0.14	−0.65–0.36	0.00	0.00	—
SoP	4	0.47	0.22–0.72	5.20	42.35	5.5	3	0.36	−0.19–0.90	15.99[a]	87.49	7.1
Total DCS	24	0.35	0.14–0.56	114.72[a]	80.12	8.2	17	0.16	−0.04–0.35	50.92[a]	68.58	15.7

Abbreviations: CBT, cognitive-behavioral therapy; CI, confidence interval; DCS, D-cycloserine; MB, methylene blue; OCD, obsessive-compulsive disorder; ORG, Org 25,935; OXT, oxytocin; PD/A, panic disorder (and/or agoraphobia); PTSD, posttraumatic stress disorder; SoP, social phobia; SpP, specific phobia; YOH, yohimbine; —, no data.

[a] $P < .05$.

there was significant heterogeneity, due to 1 of the 3 studies suggesting a small and negative effect for PAR versus PBO for CBT nonresponders with PTSD; the other 2 studies showed large positive effects for PAR in PD/A and for imipramine in depression. No follow-up data were available.

Concurrent Cognitive-Behavioral Therapy with Novel Agents

Overall, as shown in **Table 6**, the effect of novel agents versus PBO when added to CBT was small at posttreatment and at follow-up, with an NNT of 9.7 and 10.5, respectively.

Novel agents by diagnosis
No significant between-group heterogeneity was seen across diagnoses at posttreatment ($Q = 2.72, P = .74$) or at follow-up ($Q = 1.17, P = .88$), although a range of effects is noted (from $g = 0.09$ for mixed anxiety to $g = 0.41$ for SoP at posttreatment, and from $g = 0.10$ for obsessive-compulsive disorder [OCD] to $g = 0.52$ for SpP at follow-up).

Novel agents by drug
Significant between-group heterogeneity was seen across medications at posttreatment ($Q = 12.53, P = .01$) and at follow-up ($Q = 27.14, P <.001$). At posttreatment, OXT and MB were both associated with negative effects, whereas ORG, DCS, and YOH were all associated with small positive effects. At follow-up, OXT was associated with a negative effect; DCS with a negligible effect; and MB, ORG, and YOH with medium to large effects. Significant within-group heterogeneity was seen among the DCS trials, with effect sizes ranging widely from −0.93 to 1.80 at posttreatment, and from −0.59 to 1.42 at follow-up.

D-cycloserine trials by diagnosis
Because of the marked heterogeneity among the DCS trials, these studies were examined by diagnosis (**Table 6**). No significant between-diagnosis heterogeneity was found at posttreatment ($Q = 4.45, P = .49$), although significant within-diagnosis heterogeneity was seen for PTSD and SpP. Within the PTSD trials, 3 studies showed a negative effect, whereas 2 showed a large positive effect. Within the SpP trials, 1 study showed no effect, but the other 2 showed medium or large effects. At follow-up, no significant between-diagnosis heterogeneity was found ($Q = 2.53, P = .64$), although significant within-diagnosis heterogeneity was seen in OCD, PTSD, PD/A, and SoP. Follow-up effects in OCD trials ranged from −0.59 to 1.09; in PTSD trials, from −0.37 to 1.42, and in SoP trials, from −0.16 to 1.21.

SUMMARY

At this time, there is little evidence overall to suggest that antidepressant or anxiolytic medications are more efficacious than PBO when added to CBT as a first-line treatment. Although some diagnostic exceptions were noted, results did not differ significantly by diagnosis. For anxiety disorders, 9 patients need to receive additional antidepressant medications, and 18 would have to receive additional anxiolytic medications, to achieve 1 additional favorable outcome over CBT alone. For depressive disorders, 7 patients would have to receive additional antidepressant medications to achieve 1 additional favorable outcome over CBT alone.

The best cases for augmenting CBT can be made for tricyclic antidepressants, for which only 5 patients (regardless of diagnosis) would need to receive additional medications to achieve 1 additional favorable outcome over CBT alone; and GAD, for which only 3 patients would need to receive additional medications (DIA or BUS) to achieve 1 additional favorable outcome over CBT alone. However, the small number of studies in these groups precludes firm conclusions, and is overshadowed by the poor overall effects of CBT with medications over CBT + PBO.

Of note, this analysis did not consider the potential adverse effects of additive pharmacotherapy; such risks, along with the limited benefit of medications, argue against the routine administration of medications for patients with anxiety or depressive disorders receiving CBT. It is further noted that any benefits of concurrent antidepressant and anxiolytic medications with CBT are evidently lost once the medications are discontinued. Exceptions to this pattern, although statistically significant, are limited to single studies.

Although antidepressant and anxiolytic medications appear not to augment the benefits of CBT when applied concurrently, it is worth considering whether there might be subgroups of patients who are more likely to benefit from combined treatment than from CBT alone. Although several studies have investigated prognostic indicators for a specific treatment, the critical question here is of treatment moderation: patient factors that differentially predict response to combined therapy (or pharmacotherapy) versus CBT. To date, research on treatment moderation has yielded mixed results. Initial symptom severity does not differentially predict treatment outcome,[62–64] suggesting that combined treatment may not necessarily be indicated for more severe cases. The presence of comorbid personality disorder has generally not differentially influenced response to CBT versus medications,[65,66] although one study of a mixed anxious/depressed sample suggested that patients with personality disorder responded better to pharmacotherapy.[67] An emerging literature on moderating biomarkers is promising: the response of patients with OCD to medication versus CBT might be predicted by lower glucose metabolism in left orbitofrontal cortex (OFC),[68] as well as smaller gray matter volumes in right middle lateral OFC,[69] and depressed patients with hypermetabolism in parahippocampal gyrus and dorsal occipital cortex show a poorer response to CBT, but not medications.[70]

Although CBT + medications does not appear to yield benefits that are consistently superior to CBT + PBO as a first-line intervention, there is encouraging (yet sparse) evidence to support the addition of pharmacotherapy for anxious or depressed patients who fail to demonstrate an adequate response to CBT alone. Of note, this topic is seriously understudied: only 3 RCTs were found, with somewhat discrepant results and no follow-up data.

Novel agents thought to potentiate CBT mechanisms have been studied only in the anxiety disorders to date. Consistent with a recent mega-analysis demonstrating that the efficacy of DCS is small at posttreatment and negligible at follow-up,[71] in the present analysis, 7 patients would have to receive additional DCS to achieve 1 additional favorable outcome over CBT alone. It is noted that this effect is only marginally better than that of more traditional agents. Two issues have been raised regarding the benefit of DCS that merit consideration. First, some have noted that the main contribution of DCS might be to speed up the process of fear extinction; patients receiving DCS + CBT show a more rapid response than do those receiving PBO + CBT.[72,73] Thus, the benefits of DCS might be better considered from a cost-effectiveness perspective than solely from the perspective of efficacy. Second, given the working hypothesis that DCS acts on memory consolidation processes that take place after training,[74] it has been suggested that DCS would be most effective if administered judiciously, only following "successful" exposure therapy sessions. Studies in SpP[75] and SoP[76] have demonstrated that DCS appears most effective following strong within-session fear reduction, although this result was not replicated in patients with PTSD.[77]

Whereas the contribution of DCS appears to decrease over time (ie, it appears to be most effective as a treatment accelerator, is less effective at posttreatment, and is fairly ineffective at follow-up), the effects for MB and YOH follow a strikingly different pattern. These compounds' effects are fairly modest at posttreatment, but the limited available evidence suggests that these effects become stronger at follow-up. Unlike DCS, which is thought to augment CBT via potentiation of glutamatergic activity at the NMDA receptor in basolateral amygdala, MB and YOH are thought to potentiate activity in mPFC, which serves to inhibit limbic fear reactions over the course of extinction training.[39] It is possible that this different mechanism of action is more potent after treatment discontinuation, although it is noted that another compound thought to potentiate mPFC, OXT, has not been shown to have additive beneficial effects.

ACKNOWLEDGMENTS

The author thanks Dr Steven Hollon, Dr Toshi Furukawa, Amber Billingsley, and Akanksha Das for their assistance.

REFERENCES

1. Hofmann SG, Smits JA. Cognitive-behavioral therapy for adult anxiety disorders: a meta-analysis of randomized placebo-controlled trials. J Clin Psychiatry 2008; 69(4):621–32.
2. Cuijpers P, Berking M, Andersson G, et al. A meta-analysis of cognitive-behavioural therapy for adult depression, alone and in comparison with other treatments. Can J Psychiatry 2013;58(7):376–85.
3. Tolin DF. Is cognitive-behavioral therapy more effective than other therapies? A meta-analytic review. Clin Psychol Rev 2010;30(6):710–20.
4. Loerinc AG, Meuret AE, Twohig MP, et al. Response rates for CBT for anxiety disorders: need for standardized criteria. Clin Psychol Rev 2015;42:72–82.
5. Elkin I, Shea MT, Watkins JT, et al. National Institute of Mental Health Treatment of Depression Collaborative Research Program. General effectiveness of treatments. Arch Gen Psychiatry 1989;46(11):971–82 [discussion: 983].
6. Hollon SD, DeRubeis RJ, Evans MD, et al. Cognitive therapy and pharmacotherapy for depression. Singly and in combination. Arch Gen Psychiatry 1992; 49(10):774–81.
7. Rush AJ, Trivedi MH, Wisniewski SR, et al. Acute and longer-term outcomes in depressed outpatients requiring one or several treatment steps: a STAR*D report. Am J Psychiatry 2006;163(11):1905–17.
8. Turner EH, Matthews AM, Linardatos E, et al. Selective publication of antidepressant trials and its influence on apparent efficacy. N Engl J Med 2008; 358(3):252–60.
9. Jureidini JN, Doecke CJ, Mansfield PR, et al. Efficacy and safety of antidepressants for children and adolescents. BMJ 2004;328(7444):879–83.
10. Williams JW Jr, Mulrow CD, Chiquette E, et al. A systematic review of newer pharmacotherapies for depression in adults: evidence report summary. Ann Intern Med 2000;132(9):743–56.
11. Arroll B, Macgillivray S, Ogston S, et al. Efficacy and tolerability of tricyclic antidepressants and SSRIs compared with placebo for treatment of depression in primary care: a meta-analysis. Ann Fam Med 2005;3(5):449–56.
12. Undurraga J, Baldessarini RJ. Randomized, placebo-controlled trials of antidepressants for acute major depression: thirty-year meta-analytic review. Neuropsychopharmacology 2012;37(4):851–64.

13. Moncrieff J, Kirsch I. Efficacy of antidepressants in adults. BMJ 2005;331(7509): 155–7.

14. Fournier JC, DeRubeis RJ, Hollon SD, et al. Antidepressant drug effects and depression severity: a patient-level meta-analysis. JAMA 2010;303(1):47–53.

15. Kirsch I, Deacon BJ, Huedo-Medina TB, et al. Initial severity and antidepressant benefits: a meta-analysis of data submitted to the Food and Drug Administration. PLoS Med 2008;5(2):e45.

16. Bandelow B, Reitt M, Rover C, et al. Efficacy of treatments for anxiety disorders: a meta-analysis. Int Clin Psychopharmacol 2015;30(4):183–92.

17. Mitte K. Meta-analysis of cognitive-behavioral treatments for generalized anxiety disorder: a comparison with pharmacotherapy. Psychol Bull 2005;131(5): 785–95.

18. van Balkom AJ, Bakker A, Spinhoven P, et al. A meta-analysis of the treatment of panic disorder with or without agoraphobia: a comparison of psychopharmacological, cognitive-behavioral, and combination treatments. J Nerv Ment Dis 1997;185(8):510–6.

19. Abramowitz JS. Effectiveness of psychological and pharmacological treatments for obsessive-compulsive disorder: a quantitative review. J Consult Clin Psychol 1997;65(1):44–52.

20. Fedoroff IC, Taylor S. Psychological and pharmacological treatments of social phobia: a meta-analysis. J Clin Psychopharmacol 2001;21(3):311–24.

21. Imai H, Tajika A, Chen P, et al. Psychological therapies versus pharmacological interventions for panic disorder with or without agoraphobia in adults. Cochrane Database Syst Rev 2016;(10):CD011170.

22. Foa EB, Franklin ME, Moser J. Context in the clinic: how well do cognitive-behavioral therapies and medications work in combination? Biol Psychiatry 2002;52(10):987–97.

23. Otto MW, Smits JA, Reese HE. Combined psychotherapy and pharmacotherapy for mood and anxiety disorders in adults: review and analysis. Clin Psychol Sci Pract 2005;12:72–86.

24. Tolin DF. Combining pharmacotherapy and psychological treatments for OCD. In: Steketee G, editor. Oxford handbook of obsessive compulsive and spectrum disorders. New York: Oxford University Press; 2012. p. 365–75.

25. Bandelow B, Seidler-Brandler U, Becker A, et al. Meta-analysis of randomized controlled comparisons of psychopharmacological and psychological treatments for anxiety disorders. World J Biol Psychiatry 2007;8(3):175–87.

26. Furukawa TA, Watanabe N, Churchill R. Psychotherapy plus antidepressant for panic disorder with or without agoraphobia: systematic review. Br J Psychiatry 2006;188:305–12.

27. Hofmann SG, Sawyer AT, Korte KJ, et al. Is it beneficial to add pharmacotherapy to cognitive-behavioral therapy when treating anxiety disorders? A meta-analytic review. Int J Cogn Ther 2009;2(2):160–75.

28. Schweizer E, Rickels K. Placebo response in generalized anxiety: its effect on the outcome of clinical trials. J Clin Psychiatry 1997;58(Suppl 11):30–8.

29. Furukawa TA, Watanabe N, Omori IM, et al. Can pill placebo augment cognitive-behavior therapy for panic disorder? BMC Psychiatry 2007;7:73.

30. Basoglu M, Marks IM, Kilic C, et al. Alprazolam and exposure for panic disorder with agoraphobia. Attribution of improvement to medication predicts subsequent relapse. Br J Psychiatry 1994;164(5):652–9.

31. Powers MB, Smits JA, Whitley D, et al. The effect of attributional processes concerning medication taking on return of fear. J Consult Clin Psychol 2008;76(3): 478–90.
32. Kennedy WP. The nocebo reaction. Med World 1961;95:203–5.
33. Davison GC. Stepped care: doing more with less? J Consult Clin Psychol 2000; 68(4):580–5.
34. Otto MW, Pollack MH, Maki KM. Empirically supported treatments for panic disorder: costs, benefits, and stepped care. J Consult Clin Psychol 2000;68(4): 556–63.
35. Hofmann SG, Smits JA, Asnaani A, et al. Cognitive enhancers for anxiety disorders. Pharmacol Biochem Behav 2011;99(2):275–84.
36. Davis M. Role of NMDA receptors and MAP kinase in the amygdala in extinction of fear: clinical implications for exposure therapy. Eur J Neurosci 2002;16(3): 395–8.
37. Walker DL, Ressler KJ, Lu KT, et al. Facilitation of conditioned fear extinction by systemic administration or intra-amygdala infusions of D-cycloserine as assessed with fear-potentiated startle in rats. J Neurosci 2002;22(6):2343–51.
38. Nations KR, Smits JAJ, Tolin DF, et al. Evaluation of the glycine transporter inhibitor Org 25935 as augmentation to cognitive-behavioral therapy for panic disorder: A multi-center, randomized, double-blind, placebo-controlled trial. J Clin Psychiatry 2012;73:647–53.
39. Quirk GJ, Garcia R, Gonzalez-Lima F. Prefrontal mechanisms in extinction of conditioned fear. Biol Psychiatry 2006;60(4):337–43.
40. Quirk GJ, Russo GK, Barron JL, et al. The role of ventromedial prefrontal cortex in the recovery of extinguished fear. J Neurosci 2000;20(16):6225–31.
41. Milad MR, Quirk GJ. Neurons in medial prefrontal cortex signal memory for fear extinction. Nature 2002;420(6911):70–4.
42. Morris RW, Bouton ME. The effect of yohimbine on the extinction of conditioned fear: a role for context. Behav Neurosci 2007;121(3):501–14.
43. Cain CK, Blouin AM, Barad M. Adrenergic transmission facilitates extinction of conditional fear in mice. Learn Memory 2004;11(2):179–87.
44. Gonzalez-Lima F, Bruchey AK. Extinction memory improvement by the metabolic enhancer methylene blue. Learn Memory 2004;11(5):633–40.
45. Wrubel KM, Barrett D, Shumake J, et al. Methylene blue facilitates the extinction of fear in an animal model of susceptibility to learned helplessness. Neurobiol Learn Mem 2007;87(2):209–17.
46. Huber D, Veinante P, Stoop R. Vasopressin and oxytocin excite distinct neuronal populations in the central amygdala. Science 2005;308(5719):245–8.
47. Kirsch P, Esslinger C, Chen Q, et al. Oxytocin modulates neural circuitry for social cognition and fear in humans. J Neurosci 2005;25(49):11489–93.
48. American Psychiatric Association. Diagnostic and statistical manual of mental disorders. 4th text revision edition. Washington, DC: American Psychiatric Association; 2000.
49. Glass GV, McGaw B, Smith ML. Meta-analysis in social research. London: Sage Publications; 1981.
50. Borenstein M, Hedges L, Higgins J, et al. Manual: comprehensive meta-analysis software (v. 2.0). Englewood (NJ): Biostat; 2007.
51. Cohen J. Statistical power analysis for the behavioral sciences. 2nd edition. Hillsdale (NJ): Lawrence Erlbaum Associates; 1988.
52. Rosenthal R. Meta-analytic procedures for social research. London: Sage Publications; 1991.

53. Furukawa TA. From effect size into number needed to treat. Lancet 1999; 353(9165):1680.
54. Kyoto University Graduate School of Medicine/School of Public Health. EBM toolbox. 2014. Available at: http://ebmh.med.kyoto-u.ac.jp/toolbox.html. Accessed May 1, 2017.
55. Higgins JP, Thompson SG, Deeks JJ, et al. Measuring inconsistency in meta-analyses. BMJ 2003;327(7414):557–60.
56. Bartels SJ, Horn S, Sharkey P, et al. Treatment of depression in older primary care patients in health maintenance organizations. Int J Psychiatry Med 1997; 27(3):215–31.
57. Olfson M, Marcus SC, Druss B, et al. National trends in the outpatient treatment of depression. JAMA 2002;287(2):203–9.
58. Valenstein M, Taylor KK, Austin K, et al. Benzodiazepine use among depressed patients treated in mental health settings. Am J Psychiatry 2004;161(4):654–61.
59. Birkenhager TK, Moleman P, Nolen WA. Benzodiazepines for depression? A review of the literature. Int Clin Psychopharmacol 1995;10(3):181–95.
60. American Psychiatric Association. Practice guideline for the treatment of patients with major depressive disorder. Washington, DC: Author; 2010.
61. Texas medication Algorithm Project (TMAP): depression module. Austin (TX): Texas Department of Mental Health; 1998.
62. Basoglu M, Lax T, Kasvikis Y, et al. Predictors of improvement in obsessive-compulsive disorder. J Anxiety Disord 1988;2:299–317.
63. Weitz ES, Hollon SD, Twisk J, et al. Baseline depression severity as moderator of depression outcomes between cognitive behavioral therapy vs pharmacotherapy: an individual patient data meta-analysis. JAMA Psychiatry 2015; 72(11):1102–9.
64. Cuijpers P, De Wit L, Weitz E, et al. The combination of psychotherapy and pharmacotherapy in the treatment of adult depression: a comprehensive meta-analysis. J Evidence Based Psychotherap 2015;15(2):147–68.
65. Berger P, Sachs G, Amering M, et al. Personality disorder and social anxiety predict delayed response in drug and behavioral treatment of panic disorder. J Affect Disord 2004;80(1):75–8.
66. Shea MT, Pilkonis PA, Beckham E, et al. Personality disorders and treatment outcome in the NIMH Treatment of Depression Collaborative Research Program. Am J Psychiatry 1990;147(6):711–8.
67. Tyrer P, Seivewright N, Ferguson B, et al. The Nottingham study of neurotic disorder. Effect of personality status on response to drug treatment, cognitive therapy and self-help over two years. Br J Psychiatry 1993;162:219–26.
68. Brody AL, Saxena S, Schwartz JM, et al. FDG-PET predictors of response to behavioral therapy and pharmacotherapy in obsessive compulsive disorder. Psychiatry Res 1998;84(1):1–6.
69. Hoexter MQ, Dougherty DD, Shavitt RG, et al. Differential prefrontal gray matter correlates of treatment response to fluoxetine or cognitive-behavioral therapy in obsessive-compulsive disorder. Eur Neuropsychopharmacol 2013;23(7):569–80.
70. Konarski JZ, Kennedy SH, Segal ZV, et al. Predictors of nonresponse to cognitive behavioural therapy or venlafaxine using glucose metabolism in major depressive disorder. J Psychiatry Neurosci 2009;34(3):175–80.
71. Mataix-Cols D, Fernández de la Cruz F, Monzani B, et al. D-cycloserine augmentation of exposure-based cognitive-behavior therapy for anxiety, obsessive-compulsive, and posttraumatic stress disorders: Systematic review and meta-analysis of individual participant data. JAMA Psychiatry 2017;74:501–10.

72. Chasson GS, Buhlmann U, Tolin DF, et al. Need for speed: evaluating slopes of OCD recovery in behavior therapy enhanced with d-cycloserine. Behav Res Ther 2010;48(7):675–9.

73. Siegmund A, Golfels F, Finck C, et al. d-Cycloserine does not improve but might slightly speed up the outcome of in-vivo exposure therapy in patients with severe agoraphobia and panic disorder in a randomized double blind clinical trial. J Psychiatr Res 2011;45:1042–7.

74. Ledgerwood L, Richardson R, Cranney J. Effects of D-cycloserine on extinction of conditioned freezing. Behav Neurosci 2003;117(2):341–9.

75. Smits JA, Rosenfield D, Otto MW, et al. D-cycloserine enhancement of fear extinction is specific to successful exposure sessions: evidence from the treatment of height phobia. Biol Psychiatry 2013;73(11):1054–8.

76. Smits JA, Rosenfield D, Otto MW, et al. D-cycloserine enhancement of exposure therapy for social anxiety disorder depends on the success of exposure sessions. J Psychiatr Res 2013;47(10):1455–61.

77. de Kleine RA, Smits JA, Hendriks GJ, et al. Extinction learning as a moderator of d-cycloserine efficacy for enhancing exposure therapy in posttraumatic stress disorder. J Anxiety Disord 2015;34:63–7.

78. Appleby L, Warner R, Whitton A, et al. A controlled study of fluoxetine and cognitive-behavioural counselling in the treatment of postnatal depression. BMJ 1997;314(7085):932–6.

79. Barlow DH, Gorman JM, Shear MK, et al. Cognitive-behavioral therapy, imipramine, or their combination for panic disorder: a randomized controlled trial. JAMA 2000;283(19):2529–36.

80. Bellack AS, Hersen M, Himmelhoch J. Social skills training compared with pharmacotherapy and psychotherapy in the treatment of unipolar depression. Am J Psychiatry 1981;138(12):1562–7.

81. Beutler LE, Scogin F, Kirkish P, et al. Group cognitive therapy and alprazolam in the treatment of depression in older adults. J Consult Clin Psychol 1987;55(4):550–6.

82. Blomhoff S, Haug TT, Hellstrom K, et al. Randomised controlled general practice trial of sertraline, exposure therapy and combined treatment in generalised social phobia. Br J Psychiatry 2001;179:23–30.

83. Haug TT, Blomhoff S, Hellstrom K, et al. Exposure therapy and sertraline in social phobia: 1-year follow-up of a randomised controlled trial. Br J Psychiatry 2003;182:312–8.

84. Bond AJ, Wingrove J, Valerie Curran H, et al. Treatment of generalised anxiety disorder with a short course of psychological therapy, combined with buspirone or placebo. J Affect Disord 2002;72(3):267–71.

85. Chaudhry HR, Najam N, Naqvi A. The value of amineptine in depressed patients treated with cognitive behavioural psychotherapy. Hum Psychopharmacol 1998;13:419–24.

86. Clark DM, Ehlers A, McManus F, et al. Cognitive therapy versus fluoxetine in generalized social phobia: a randomized placebo-controlled trial. J Consult Clin Psychol 2003;71(6):1058–67.

87. Cohen JA, Mannarino AP, Perel JM, et al. A pilot randomized controlled trial of combined trauma-focused CBT and sertraline for childhood PTSD symptoms. J Am Acad Child Adolesc Psychiatry 2007;46(7):811–9.

88. Cottraux J, Mollard E, Bouvard M, et al. A controlled study of fluvoxamine and exposure in obsessive-compulsive disorder. Int Clin Psychopharmacol 1990;5(1):17–30.

89. Cottraux J, Mollard E, Bouvard M, et al. Exposure therapy, fluvoxamine, or combination treatment in obsessive-compulsive disorder: one-year followup. Psychiatry Res 1993;49(1):63–75.
90. Cottraux J, Note ID, Cungi C, et al. A controlled study of cognitive behaviour therapy with buspirone or placebo in panic disorder with agoraphobia. Br J Psychiatry 1995;167(5):635–41.
91. Davidson JR, Foa EB, Huppert JD, et al. Fluoxetine, comprehensive cognitive behavioral therapy, and placebo in generalized social phobia. Arch Gen Psychiatry 2004;61(10):1005–13.
92. de Beurs E, van Balkom AJ, Lange A, et al. Treatment of panic disorder with agoraphobia: comparison of fluvoxamine, placebo, and psychological panic management combined with exposure and of exposure in vivo alone. Am J Psychiatry 1995;152(5):683–91.
93. de Beurs E, van Balkom AJ, Van Dyck R, et al. Long-term outcome of pharmacological and psychological treatment for panic disorder with agoraphobia: a 2-year naturalistic follow-up. Acta Psychiatr Scand 1999;99(1):59–67.
94. Echeburua E, De Corral P, Bajos EG, et al. Interactions between self-exposure and alprazolam in the treatment of agoraphobia without panic: an exploratory study. Behav Cogn Psychother 1993;21:219–38.
95. Fahy TJ, O'Rourke D, Brophy J, et al. The Galway Study of Panic Disorder. I: Clomipramine and lofepramine in DSM III-R panic disorder: a placebo controlled trial. J Affect Disord 1992;25(1):63–75.
96. Gingnell M, Frick A, Engman J, et al. Combining escitalopram and cognitive-behavioural therapy for social anxiety disorder: randomised controlled fMRI trial. Br J Psychiatry 2016;209(3):229–35.
97. Hohagen F, Winkelmann G, Rasche-Ruchle H, et al. Combination of behaviour therapy with fluvoxamine in comparison with behaviour therapy and placebo. Results of a multicentre study. Br J Psychiatry 1998;35:71–8.
98. Loerch B, Graf-Morgenstern M, Hautzinger M, et al. Randomised placebo-controlled trial of moclobemide, cognitive-behavioural therapy and their combination in panic disorder with agoraphobia. Br J Psychiatry 1999;174:205–12.
99. Marks IM, Gray S, Cohen D, et al. Imipramine and brief therapist-aided exposure in agoraphobics having self-exposure homework. Arch Gen Psychiatry 1983;40(2):153–62.
100. Murphy GE, Simons AD, Wetzel RD, et al. Cognitive therapy and pharmacotherapy. Singly and together in the treatment of depression. Arch Gen Psychiatry 1984;41(1):33–41.
101. Simons AD, Murphy GE, Levine JL, et al. Cognitive therapy and pharmacotherapy for depression. Sustained improvement over one year. Arch Gen Psychiatry 1986;43(1):43–8.
102. Peter H, Tabrizian S, Hand I. Serum cholesterol in patients with obsessive compulsive disorder during treatment with behavior therapy and SSRI or placebo. Int J Psychiatry Med 2000;30(1):27–39.
103. Power KG, Simpson RJ, Swanson V, et al. A controlled comparison of cognitive-behaviour therapy, diazepam, and placebo, alone and in combination, for the treatment of generalised anxiety disorder. J Anxiety Disord 1990;4:267–92.
104. Ravindran AV, Anisman H, Merali Z, et al. Treatment of primary dysthymia with group cognitive therapy and pharmacotherapy: clinical symptoms and functional impairments. Am J Psychiatry 1999;156(10):1608–17.
105. Roth WT, Telch MJ, Taylor CB, et al. Autonomic changes after treatment of agoraphobia with panic attacks. Psychiatry Res 1987;24:95–107.

106. Rothbaum BO, Price M, Jovanovic T, et al. A randomized, double-blind evaluation of D-cycloserine or alprazolam combined with virtual reality exposure therapy for posttraumatic stress disorder in Iraq and Afghanistan War veterans. Am J Psychiatry 2014;171(6):640–8.

107. Schneier FR, Neria Y, Pavlicova M, et al. Combined prolonged exposure therapy and paroxetine for PTSD related to the World Trade Center attack: a randomized controlled trial. Am J Psychiatry 2012;169(1):80–8.

108. Sharp DM, Power KG, Simpson RJ, et al. Fluvoxamine, placebo, and cognitive behaviour therapy used alone and in combination in the treatment of panic disorder and agoraphobia. J Anxiety Disord 1996;10(4):219–42.

109. Stein MB, Norton GR, Walker JR, et al. Do selective serotonin re-uptake inhibitors enhance the efficacy of very brief cognitive behavioral therapy for panic disorder? A pilot study. Psychiatry Res 2000;94(3):191–200.

110. Storch EA, Bussing R, Small BJ, et al. Randomized, placebo-controlled trial of cognitive-behavioral therapy alone or combined with sertraline in the treatment of pediatric obsessive-compulsive disorder. Behav Res Ther 2013;51(12): 823–9.

111. Telch MJ, Agras WS, Taylor CB, et al. Combined pharmacological and behavioral treatment for agoraphobia. Behav Res Ther 1985;23(3):325–35.

112. Wardle J, Hayward P, Higgitt A, et al. Effects of concurrent diazepam treatment on the outcome of exposure therapy in agoraphobia. Behav Res Ther 1994; 32(2):203–15.

113. Wilson PH. Combined pharmacological and behavioural treatment of depression. Behav Res Ther 1982;20(2):173–84.

114. Simon NM, Connor KM, Lang AJ, et al. Paroxetine CR augmentation for posttraumatic stress disorder refractory to prolonged exposure therapy. J Clin Psychiatry 2008;69(3):400–5.

115. Kampman M, Keijsers GP, Hoogduin CA, et al. A randomized, double-blind, placebo-controlled study of the effects of adjunctive paroxetine in panic disorder patients unsuccessfully treated with cognitive-behavioral therapy alone. J Clin Psychiatry 2002;63(9):772–7.

116. Stewart JW, Mercier MA, Agosti V, et al. Imipramine is effective after unsuccessful cognitive therapy: sequential use of cognitive therapy and imipramine in depressed outpatients. J Clin Psychopharmacol 1993;13(2):114–9.

117. Acheson DT, Feifel D, Kamenski M, et al. Intranasal oxytocin administration prior to exposure therapy for arachnophobia impedes treatment response. Depress Anxiety 2015;32(6):400–7.

118. Andersson E, Hedman E, Enander J, et al. D-cycloserine vs placebo as adjunct to cognitive behavioral therapy for obsessive-compulsive disorder and interaction with antidepressants: a randomized clinical trial. JAMA Psychiatry 2015; 72(7):659–67.

119. de Kleine RA, Hendriks GJ, Kusters WJ, et al. A randomized placebo-controlled trial of D-cycloserine to enhance exposure therapy for posttraumatic stress disorder. Biol Psychiatry 2012;71(11):962–8.

120. Difede J, Cukor J, Wyka K, et al. D-cycloserine augmentation of exposure therapy for post-traumatic stress disorder: a pilot randomized clinical trial. Neuropsychopharmacology 2014;39(5):1052–8.

121. Farrell LJ, Waters AM, Boschen MJ, et al. Difficult-to-treat pediatric obsessive-compulsive disorder: feasibility and preliminary results of a randomized pilot trial of D-cycloserine-augmented behavior therapy. Depress Anxiety 2013;30(8): 723–31.

122. Guastella AJ, Richardson R, Lovibond PF, et al. A randomized controlled trial of D-cycloserine enhancement of exposure therapy for social anxiety disorder. Biol Psychiatry 2008;63(6):544–9.

123. Guastella AJ, Howard AL, Dadds MR, et al. A randomized controlled trial of intranasal oxytocin as an adjunct to exposure therapy for social anxiety disorder. Psychoneuroendocrinology 2009;34(6):917–23.

124. Hofmann SG, Meuret AE, Smits JA, et al. Augmentation of exposure therapy with D-cycloserine for social anxiety disorder. Arch Gen Psychiatry 2006;63(3): 298–304.

125. Hofmann SG, Smits JA, Rosenfield D, et al. D-cycloserine as an augmentation strategy with cognitive-behavioral therapy for social anxiety disorder. Am J Psychiatry 2013;170:751–8.

126. Kushner MG, Kim SW, Donahue C, et al. D-cycloserine augmented exposure therapy for obsessive-compulsive disorder. Biol Psychiatry 2007;62(8):835–8.

127. Litz BT, Salters-Pedneault K, Steenkamp MM, et al. A randomized placebo-controlled trial of D-cycloserine and exposure therapy for posttraumatic stress disorder. J Psychiatr Res 2012;46(9):1184–90.

128. Mataix-Cols D, Turner C, Monzani B, et al. Cognitive-behavioural therapy with post-session D-cycloserine augmentation for paediatric obsessive-compulsive disorder: pilot randomised controlled trial. Br J Psychiatry 2014;204(1):77–8.

129. Meyerbroeker K, Powers MB, van Stegeren A, et al. Does yohimbine hydrochloride facilitate fear extinction in virtual reality treatment of fear of flying? A randomized placebo-controlled trial. Psychother Psychosom 2012;81(1):29–37.

130. Nave AM, Tolin DF, Stevens MC. Exposure therapy, D-cycloserine, and functional magnetic resonance imaging in patients with snake phobia: a randomized pilot study. J Clin Psychiatry 2012;73(9):1179–86.

131. Otto MW, Tolin DF, Simon NM, et al. Efficacy of d-cycloserine for enhancing response to cognitive-behavior therapy for panic disorder. Biol Psychiatry 2010;67(4):365–70.

132. Otto MW, Pollack MH, Dowd SM, et al. Randomized trial of d-cycloserine enhancement of cognitive-behavioral therapy for panic disorder. Depress Anxiety 2016;33(8):737–45.

133. Powers MB, Smits JA, Otto MW, et al. Facilitation of fear extinction in phobic participants with a novel cognitive enhancer: a randomized placebo controlled trial of yohimbine augmentation. J Anxiety Disord 2009;23(3):350–6.

134. Ressler KJ, Rothbaum BO, Tannenbaum L, et al. Cognitive enhancers as adjuncts to psychotherapy: use of D-cycloserine in phobic individuals to facilitate extinction of fear. Arch Gen Psychiatry 2004;61(11):1136–44.

135. Rapee RM, Jones MP, Hudson JL, et al. D-cycloserine does not enhance the effects of in vivo exposure among young people with broad-based anxiety disorders. Behav Res Ther 2016;87:225–31.

136. Scheeringa MS, Weems CF. Randomized placebo-controlled D-cycloserine with cognitive behavior therapy for pediatric posttraumatic stress. J Child Adolesc Psychopharmacol 2014;24(2):69–77.

137. Smits JA, Rosenfield D, Davis ML, et al. Yohimbine enhancement of exposure therapy for social anxiety disorder: a randomized controlled trial. Biol Psychiatry 2014;75(11):840–6.

138. Storch EA, Merlo LJ, Bengtson M, et al. D-cycloserine does not enhance exposure-response prevention therapy in obsessive-compulsive disorder. Int Clin Psychopharmacol 2007;22(4):230–7.

139. Storch EA, Murphy TK, Goodman WK, et al. A preliminary study of D-cycloserine augmentation of cognitive-behavioral therapy in pediatric obsessive-compulsive disorder. Biol Psychiatry 2010;68(11):1073–6.
140. Storch EA, Wilhelm S, Sprich S, et al. Efficacy of augmentation of cognitive behavior therapy with weight-adjusted d-cycloserine vs placebo in pediatric obsessive-compulsive disorder: a randomized clinical trial. JAMA Psychiatry 2016;73(8):779–88.
141. Tart CD, Handelsman PR, Deboer LB, et al. Augmentation of exposure therapy with post-session administration of D-cycloserine. J Psychiatr Res 2013;47(2): 168–74.
142. Telch MJ, Bruchey AK, Rosenfield D, et al. Effects of post-session administration of methylene blue on fear extinction and contextual memory in adults with claustrophobia. Am J Psychiatry 2014;171(10):1091–8.
143. Wilhelm S, Buhlmann U, Tolin DF, et al. Augmentation of behavior therapy with D-cycloserine for obsessive-compulsive disorder. Am J Psychiatry 2008; 165(3):335–41.
144. Zoellner LA, Telch M, Foa EB, et al. Enhancing extinction learning in posttraumatic stress disorder with brief daily imaginal exposure and methylene blue: a randomized controlled trial. J Clin Psychiatry 2017;78(7):e782–9.

Mindfulness-Based Interventions for Anxiety and Depression

Stefan G. Hofmann, PhD*, Angelina F. Gómez, BA

KEYWORDS

- Mindfulness • Mindfulness-based interventions • Anxiety • Depression
- Cognitive behavior therapy

KEY POINTS

- Research on mindfulness-based interventions (MBIs) for anxiety and depression has increased rapidly in the past decade. The most common include mindfulness-based stress reduction and mindfulness-based cognitive therapy.
- MBIs have shown efficacy in reducing anxiety and depression symptom severity in a broad range of treatment-seeking individuals.
- MBIs consistently outperform non–evidence-based treatments and active control conditions, such as health education, relaxation training, and supportive psychotherapy.
- MBIs also perform comparably with cognitive behavior therapy (CBT). The treatment principles of MBIs for anxiety and depression are compatible with those of standard CBT.

INTRODUCTION

Buddhist traditions first explored the concept of mindfulness in broad philosophic terms unfamiliar to most modern readers. Nevertheless, mindfulness has spread rapidly in Western psychology research and practice, in large part because of the success of standardized mindfulness-based interventions.[1] These interventions, namely mindfulness-based stress reduction (MBSR)[2] and mindfulness-based cognitive therapy (MBCT),[3] incorporate the essence of Eastern mindfulness practices into Western cognitive-behavioral practice. The body of literature on mindfulness-based interventions (MBIs) has grown rapidly in recent years.[4,5] Despite the popularity of these interventions, the evidence base is still not fully established, in part because this literature contains many cross-sectional studies, waitlist-controlled trials, and other methodological shortcomings that limit the strength of conclusions that can be drawn from these studies.[1] Considering these weaknesses, clinical researchers have increasingly

Disclosure: The authors have nothing to disclose.
Department of Psychological and Brain Sciences, Boston University, 648 Beacon Street, 6th Floor, Boston, MA 02215, USA
* Corresponding author.
E-mail address: shofmann@bu.edu

Psychiatr Clin N Am 40 (2017) 739–749
http://dx.doi.org/10.1016/j.psc.2017.08.008
0193-953X/17/© 2017 Elsevier Inc. All rights reserved.

psych.theclinics.com

studied MBIs with more rigorous methodology, allowing select meaningful conclusions to be drawn from the present body of work.

Recent reviews of well-designed randomized controlled trials comparing mindfulness treatments (primarily MBSR and MBCT) with active control conditions indicate that MBIs are effective in treating a broad range of outcomes among diverse populations.[6-11] These outcomes include clinical disorders and symptoms such as anxiety,[8,12,13] risk of relapse for depression,[14,15] current depressive symptoms,[9] stress,[16-18] medical and well-being outcomes such as chronic pain,[19] quality of life,[14,20] and psychological or emotional distress.[21,22] In addition, MBIs have been shown to work via changes in specific aspects of mental disorder, such as cognitive biases, affective dysregulation, and interpersonal effectiveness.[17,23,24]

In addition to the mindfulness-based treatment protocols, mindfulness principles have been integrated into other notable therapeutic interventions such as dialectical behavioral therapy (DBT)[25] and acceptance and commitment therapy (ACT).[26] In addition, mindfulness has increasingly been explored within the context of cognitive behavior therapy (CBT) for emotional disorders.[27] The use of mindfulness in these treatment protocols is markedly different from MBSR and MBCT, in that mindfulness is merely a component of these interventions, whereas it is the core skill taught in mindfulness-based treatments. In addition, these treatments include other, nonmindfulness therapeutic ingredients, thus making it difficult to attribute therapeutic effects to mindfulness skills specifically.[1,28] Despite these distinctions, MBIs are compatible with the dominant cognitive behavior psychotherapy practiced today. CBT is an umbrella term that refers to a conceptual model of treatment more than any single protocol.[29,30] Mindfulness and acceptance strategies are consistent with general CBT principles because they target core processes, such as increased emotional awareness and regulation, cognitive flexibility, and goals-based behaviors.[31,32] This topic is outside the boundaries of this article but it is likely to become part of the future of psychotherapy. As discussed throughout this article, mindfulness targets one such core process that has shown efficacy in reducing anxiety and depression symptom severity, as the core treatment ingredient as well as when integrated into other treatments. The primary aim of this article is to explore the ways in which cognitive and behavioral treatments for depression and anxiety have been advanced by the application of mindfulness practices.

OVERVIEW OF MINDFULNESS TREATMENTS

The overarching theoretic premise of MBIs is that, by practicing mindfulness (eg, through sitting meditation, yoga, or other mindfulness exercises), individuals become less reactive to unpleasant internal phenomena but more reflective, which in turn leads to positive psychological outcomes.[3,33] This article briefly reviews the most recent literature in mindfulness-based treatments for anxiety and depression, starting with current perspectives in the definition and measurement of mindfulness.

What is Mindfulness?

Mindfulness refers to a process that leads to a mental state characterized by nonjudgmental awareness of the present moment experience, including the person's sensations, thoughts, bodily states, consciousness, and the environment, while encouraging openness, curiosity, and acceptance.[34-36] Bishop and colleagues[34] (2004) distinguished 2 components of mindfulness, 1 that involves self-regulation of attention and 1 that involves an orientation toward the present moment characterized by curiosity, openness, and acceptance.

Mindfulness stands in stark contrast with much of people's common daily experience, because the default mode of attention for many individuals is nonattention. Mind wandering is ubiquitous,[37] as is the state of mindlessly going through daily activities, often known as running on autopilot."[38] When people do manage to focus on internal experiences in the present moment, this attention is often filled with self-critical, ruminative, or otherwise worrisome thoughts and emotions that people then attempt to suppress.[39] The experience of attending to the present moment can be so aversive that some people prefer almost anything else; a review of 11 laboratory studies with healthy adults found that most people choose to do mundane tasks, or even receive mild electric shocks, rather than be left alone with their own thoughts.[40]

Despite their predominance in daily life, mindless states have been shown to be maladaptive. In a large study using ecological momentary assessment data,[37] approximately 47% of subjects' waking hours were spent in a state of mind wandering; furthermore, the investigators showed that mind wandering predicts subsequent unhappiness. In contrast, the capacity to keep the mind focused on the present moment is associated with higher psychological well-being.[41] Taken together, these findings suggest that mindfulness is a difficult state to achieve but is ultimately beneficial. This skill has been likened to the cognitive science theory of a desirable difficulty, which is essentially a task that requires expenditure of cognitive resources but results in higher cognitive flexibility, insight, and self-regulation abilities.[4]

Mindfulness is thus both a skill and a practice; the practice of mindfulness begets the skill of staying mindful. The stronger the ability to adopt a mindful state throughout the perpetual ups and downs of life, the less suffering will be experienced. This basic premise remains the foundation of mindful practices, as it has for centuries[42]; however, when clinical scientists attempt to parse apart the mechanisms of this seemingly simple process, the evidence rapidly becomes messy and ill-defined. Whichever mechanisms truly underlie mindfulness (key mechanisms are reviewed later), mindfulness practices seem to show therapeutic effects on emotional well-being, and thus continue to capture the interest of myriad clients, practitioners, and researchers.

Mindfulness-based Stress Reduction

The first and perhaps the most well-known mindfulness-based intervention to gain empirical support in the treatment of psychological symptoms is MBSR, developed by Jon Kabat-Zinn[2] in the early 1980s. MBSR is an 8-week treatment program that is designed to reduce stress via enhanced mindfulness skills developed through regular meditation practices. The program consists of weekly 2-hour to 2.5-hour group-based meditation classes with a trained teacher, daily audio-guided home practice (approximately 45 min/d), and a day-long mindfulness retreat occurring during the sixth week. Much of the course content is focused on learning how to mindfully attend to body sensations, using various mind-body meditative practices such as sitting meditation, body scans, gentle stretching, and yoga. In addition, the group classes foster discussion of how to apply these mindful practices in daily life, with the ultimate effect of being able to handle stressors in a more adaptive way. The MBSR program was initially developed to treat medical patients with chronic pain[2] but has since been applied to many other populations of medical and psychiatric patients, as well as community members.[43] Across these various groups, MBSR has consistently been found to be tolerable, with high rates of compliance, program completion, and patient satisfaction.[6,44,45]

Studies comparing MBSR with active control conditions have shown that MBIs are superior in reducing anxiety symptoms. Hoge and colleagues[46] found that MBSR outperformed an active stress-management education program in a group of individuals with generalized anxiety disorder. More specifically, individuals in the MBSR group showed significantly more reduction in anxiety symptom severity than the control group, as measured by self-report measures of anxiety as well as anxiety in response to a laboratory social stress challenge task. The MBSR group showed a pretreatment-posttreatment effect size (Cohen d) of 1.06, which is comparable with the effect sizes seen in CBT for anxiety. These results are supported by select meta-analyses that have shown the superiority of MBSR in reducing anxiety and stress relative to heterogeneous control conditions.[8,47,48] Pretreatment-posttreatment treatment effect sizes for these meta-analyses are all in the moderate to large range (Hedges g from 0.24–1.54).

MBSR seems to be a safe and effective treatment to reduce emotional dysregulation. In addition, researchers have adapted the many basic principles of the program into modified protocols to treat specific populations and outcomes. These principles include MBCT for depression,[15] mindfulness-based relapse prevention for drug addiction,[49] mindfulness-based relationship enhancement to improve relationship functioning,[50] and a mindfulness-based program to foster healthy eating.[51]

Mindfulness-based Cognitive Therapy

The most widely researched adaptation of MBSR is MBCT, originally developed by Teasdale and colleagues[15] to prevent relapse of major depression. As its name implies, MBCT combines elements of both mindfulness training and cognitive therapy to reduce the recurrence of depression. Mindfulness principles are applied to aid individuals in recognizing deterioration of mood without immediately judging or reacting to this change. This enhanced internal awareness is then combined with principles of cognitive therapy that teach individuals to disengage from maladaptive patterns of repetitive negative thinking that contribute to depressive symptoms.[52] Other than this additional cognitive therapy component, MBCT closely follows the structure of MBSR, including the 8-week group-based format, and the length and type of homework assignments.

Since its initial development, several well-designed randomized controlled trials examining the efficacy of MBCT relative to control conditions have shown that the program is effective in reducing rates of relapse among individuals with major depression.[4] Furthermore, studies of individual moderators of treatment outcomes have found that MBCT may be most effective in preventing relapse among individuals with the greatest risk of relapse. These high-risk individuals include those with 4 or more previous major depressive episodes (Cohen $h = 0.88$),[53] and those who experienced maltreatment during childhood.[53,54] In addition to preventing rates of relapse, MBCT has also shown efficacy in reducing current acute depression symptoms (Hedges $g = 0.73$).[9]

In one of these trials, Eisendrath and colleagues[55] tested the efficacy of a modified MBCT program for individuals with current treatment-resistant depression. MBCT reduced depressive symptoms posttreatment compared with a well-matched active control program (health enhancement program). Despite these promising findings, the MBCT and control groups did not differ significantly on rates of depression remission, suggesting that the effects of MBCT were not strong enough to achieve full disorder remission. These findings also show the importance of a well-matched control condition. Until recent years, most trials compared MBIs with waitlist controls, which introduce a multitude of confounding factors that limit the strength of conclusions that can be drawn from these trials. Given that MBCT was no better than a general health education program in achieving depression remission in this high-quality trial, the results of waitlist-controlled trials should be interpreted with great caution.

Other Mindfulness-based Treatments

MBSR and MBCT are intensive treatment programs requiring a sizable commitment in terms of both patient and therapist time and training. In addition to these standardized treatments, mindfulness practices have been applied therapeutically in several other ways.

Retreats and residential programs
One popular treatment delivery method is mindfulness meditation retreats, which typically range from 1 to 3 days but can extend for as long as 3 months.[4] These retreats vary greatly in terms of their format and target population, and there is scant research on their short-term and long-term effects. Nevertheless, these retreats are a fairly cost-effective way of delivering intensive and well-controlled doses of a mindfulness intervention, and recent trials have shown promising effects on anxiety, stress, and other measures of psychosocial well-being and health.[56,57]

Brief mindfulness interventions
Some investigators have adapted the MBSR treatment protocol into abbreviated programs of 2 to 3 weeks.[58,59] These programs have not been examined as thoroughly as the standard 8-week interventions; however, preliminary evidence indicates that these modest interventions can have beneficial effects on a variety of symptoms, including compassion[58] and working memory capacity.[59] It is as yet unclear whether these abbreviated mindfulness interventions can effectively reduce clinical levels of anxiety or depression, although the potential for beneficial effects in a fraction of the time warrants further study.

Another emerging adaptation of standard MBIs is even shorter, 3-day or 4-day, laboratory-based mindfulness training.[60] These brief and highly controlled interventions typically involve 20-minute to 30-minute group sessions conducted by a trained meditation instructor, and minimal to no required practice outside of the laboratory.[61] Although these mindfulness interventions are too truncated to provide any long-term effects, studies indicate that they can have immediate effects on psychological and neuroendocrine responses to social stress,[60] as well as perceived pain severity in response to noxious heat stimulation.[61] These significant effects after only a few days of mindfulness training are exciting, and future research should explore whether such brief interventions can have similar effects on symptoms of anxiety or depression. Regardless, these shorter mindfulness interventions offer 1 clear benefit already, in that they afford greater research flexibility to conduct both efficacy-focused and mechanisms-focused trials.[4]

Internet and smartphone mindfulness-based interventions
Another new development in the mindfulness literature is the recent surge of Internet-based and app-based MBIs. These interventions vary a great deal in treatment length, ranging from 8-week programs that closely mimic the MBSR protocol[62] to 2-week or 3-week self-guided interventions with little formal structure.[58,63] Although these technology-delivered interventions are still in their infancy, a recent meta-analysis of 15 randomized controlled trials found that, relative to control or waitlist conditions, technology-delivered MBIs had a significant beneficial impact on depression, anxiety, stress, well-being, and mindfulness (Hedges g ranging from 0.22 for anxiety to 0.51 for stress).[64] Although studies have not yet examined the efficacy of online MBIs

compared with in-person approaches, these preliminary findings are promising and warrant further research.

Summary: Efficacy of Mindfulness-based Interventions for Anxiety and Depression

Randomized controlled trials comparing MBSR with active control conditions indicate that MBSR is moderately to largely effective at reducing anxiety and depression symptom severity among individuals with a broad range of medical and psychiatric conditions. The most comprehensive review to date[6] examined the effects of 209 trials of MBIs among 12,145 patients with a variety of disorders. The results indicated that MBIs are more effective in reducing psychological and medical symptom severity than waitlist, psychoeducation, supportive psychotherapy, relaxation training, and imagery or suppression techniques. Posttreatment effect sizes were largest for psychological outcomes, relative to physical or medical outcomes, with the strongest effects found for anxiety, followed by depression. These beneficial effects remained fairly stable after follow-up periods (ranging from 3 weeks to 3 years, with a median of 28 weeks), although the comparative effect sizes for MBI versus control treatment conditions diminished at follow-up.[6] Collectively, these results indicate that MBIs are more effective than non–evidence-based treatments in reducing anxiety and depression symptom severity among a broad range of treatment-seeking individuals. However, as noted by Dimidjian and Segal,[65] there have been several methodological gaps that restrict both the reach and relevance of the conclusions that can be drawn from the current literature.

MINDFULNESS IN THE CONTEXT OF COGNITIVE BEHAVIOR THERAPY

Mindfulness-based treatments and traditional (beckian) CBT share many similar characteristics.[45] Both aim to reduce psychopathologic suffering, and approach this goal with a combination of cognitive and behavioral therapeutic exercises. Both involve a desensitization of conditioned fear responses, although MBIs approach this effect through sustained attention, whereas traditional CBT directly focuses on severing the conditioned response through exposure-based processes.[66] Another key similarity between traditional CBT and MBIs is the directive for patients to view their internal phenomena (thoughts, feelings, sensations) as temporary and without inherent worth or meaning. Again, MBIs approach this process through simple observation, whereas traditional CBT involves directly challenging metacognitions about such phenomena.[67] In addition, both treatments involve relaxation and improvements in self-modulatory efforts,[45] although it is unclear whether these effects are attributable to a specific treatment component or simply engaging in a therapeutic process.

There are also key differences between mindfulness interventions and traditional CBT. Perhaps the most evident difference is the focus on accepting versus changing maladaptive cognitions. Although traditional CBT includes elements of both these directives, the overall aim of traditional CBT is to challenge automatic thoughts by holding them up to disconfirming evidence, and then to change them into different thoughts.[68] This cognitive restructuring process is antithetical to mindfulness principles, which encourage a complete lack of engagement with cognitive and emotional processes. Another key distinction is the degree to which each treatment is goal oriented. CBT typically begins with the client identifying the primary treatment goals (eg, improve mood, reduce maladaptive behaviors), and continues helping the client to strive toward these goals. Although clients seek mindfulness-based treatments for similar reasons, the therapeutic process involves little attention to such goals, instead cultivating a seemingly paradoxic attitude of nonstriving.[45]

Despite these differences, the result of both approaches is ultimately similar: by changing the patient's perspective on unpleasant thoughts, feelings, or sensations, the individual comes to realize that these internal phenomena are not as dangerous or powerful as previously thought, and the cycle of maladaptive cognitions, emotions, and behaviors gradually weakens. These similarities may be responsible for the compatibility of mindfulness and cognitive-behavioral treatments.

Mindfulness as a Component of Cognitive-Behavioral Treatments

Before the widespread interest in mindfulness-specific treatments, mindfulness was included as a component of broader evidence-based interventions, such as DBT, ACT, cognitive behavioral stress management, and integrative body-mind training.[4] Although these treatments focus on disparate clinical populations and symptoms, efficacy evidence for each suggests that mindfulness training is a key beneficial component of these interventions.[69] This article briefly reviews the 2 most common therapies (DBT and ACT) and the role that mindfulness plays in each.

Dialectical behavior therapy

DBT was developed by Marsha Linehan[25] for the treatment of individuals with borderline personality disorder. This multifaceted intervention is founded on the concept of a unified dialectic; essentially, the view that life is composed of opposing forces that must be simultaneously accepted to achieve beneficial change. Mindfulness is taught as a skill to help clients recognize and synthesize the key dialectic; namely the contrast between acceptance and change. Mindfulness skills taught in DBT are similar to those in MBSR, particularly the nonjudgmental observation of internal phenomena; however, the format in which these skills are taught differs considerably. Unlike MBSR, which prescribes a specific dose of meditative practice, mindfulness training is one of many skills taught throughout a year-long weekly skills group (other skills include interpersonal effectiveness, emotion regulation, and distress tolerance). In addition, clients learn mindfulness through numerous exercises, rather than predominantly through meditation as in MBSR. These exercises include imagery practices (eg, imagining that the mind is a conveyor belt), breath-focused exercises (eg, breath counting, coordinating breaths with footsteps), and various other exercises that encourage clients to practice mindfulness throughout daily tasks such as showering or doing the dishes.[25,45] Clients may choose which mindfulness exercises they wish to practice and when, which allows all individuals to benefit from mindfulness training regardless of their severity or willingness to meditate.[45]

Acceptance and commitment therapy

ACT was developed by Hayes and Wilson[26] as a contemporary approach to general adult outpatient psychotherapy based in classic behavior-analytical principles. ACT does not include meditation practices and rarely uses the term mindfulness in its treatment protocol, but the therapeutic strategies of ACT are practically identical to mindfulness skills as described in this article. For example, a core principle of ACT is the observing self, in which clients cultivate the ability to simply observe internal phenomena, without attaching to, evaluating, or attempting to change them. Clients attempt to see themselves as separate from their distressing thoughts, feelings, and sensations, and are encouraged to accept such phenomena as they are, while changing maladaptive behaviors to improve their lives.[26,45]

SUMMARY

Mindfulness-based and acceptance-based interventions, including DBT, ACT, MBSR, and MBCT, are examples of the so-called third wave of CBTs.[70] After a contentious debate about the meaning, validity, and relevance of the term third wave,[4,29] 2 prominent representatives from both camps (Steven Hayes and Stefan Hofmann, who is also the first author of this article), recently joined forces based on the evidence and their shared beliefs and values. The result is a call to redirect clinical practice away from treating medical syndromes and toward focusing on processes and core competencies. MBIs target one such process. A more detailed discussion of this can be found elsewhere.[31,32]

REFERENCES

1. Gu J, Strauss C, Bond R, et al. How do mindfulness-based cognitive therapy and mindfulness-based stress reduction improve mental health and wellbeing? A systematic review and meta-analysis of mediation studies. Clin Psychol Rev 2015;37: 1–12.
2. Kabat-Zinn J. An outpatient program in behavioral medicine for chronic pain patients based on the practice of mindfulness meditation: theoretical considerations and preliminary results. Gen Hosp Psychiatry 1982;4(1):33–47.
3. Segal ZV, Williams JMG, Teasdale JD. Mindfulness-based cognitive therapy for depression: a new approach to preventing relapse. New York: Guilford Press; 2002.
4. Creswell JD. Mindfulness interventions. Annu Rev Psychol 2017;68:491–516.
5. Hofmann SG, Asmundson GJG. Acceptance and mindfulness-based therapy: new wave or old hat? Clin Psychol Rev 2008;28(1):1–16.
6. Khoury B, Lecomte T, Fortin G, et al. Mindfulness-based therapy: a comprehensive meta-analysis. Clin Psychol Rev 2013;33(6):763–71.
7. Eberth J, Sedlmeier P. The effects of mindfulness meditation: a meta-analysis. Mindfulness 2012;3(3):174–89.
8. Hofmann SG, Sawyer AT, Witt AA, et al. The effect of mindfulness-based therapy on anxiety and depression: a meta-analytic review. J Consult Clin Psychol 2010; 78(2):169–83.
9. Strauss C, Cavanagh K, Oliver A, et al. Mindfulness-based interventions for people diagnosed with a current episode of an anxiety or depressive disorder: a meta-analysis of randomised controlled trials. PLoS One 2014;9(4):e96110.
10. Piet J, Hougaard E. The effect of mindfulness-based cognitive therapy for prevention of relapse in recurrent major depressive disorder: a systematic review and meta-analysis. Clin Psychol Rev 2011;31(6):1032–40.
11. Goyal M, Singh S, Sibinga EMS, et al. Meditation programs for psychological stress and well-being: a systematic review and meta-analysis. JAMA Intern Med 2014;174(3):357–68.
12. Green SM, Bieling PJ. Expanding the scope of mindfulness-based cognitive therapy: evidence for effectiveness in a heterogeneous psychiatric sample. Cogn Behav Pract. http://dx.doi.org/10.1016/j.cbpra.2011.02.006.
13. Hinton DE, Pich V, Hofmann SG, et al. Acceptance and mindfulness techniques as applied to refugee and ethnic minority populations with PTSD: examples from "culturally adapted CBT". Cogn Behav Pract 2013;20(1):33–46.
14. Kuyken W, Byford S, Taylor RS, et al. Mindfulness-based cognitive therapy to prevent relapse in recurrent depression. J Consult Clin Psychol 2008;76(6):966–78.

15. Teasdale JD, Segal ZV, Williams JMG, et al. Prevention of relapse/recurrence in major depression by mindfulness-based cognitive therapy. J Consult Clin Psychol 2000;68(4):615–23.

16. Chiesa A, Serretti A. Mindfulness-based stress reduction for stress management in healthy people: a review and meta-analysis. J Altern Complement Med 2009; 15(5):593–600.

17. Bullis JR, Boe HJ, Asnaani A, et al. The benefits of being mindful: trait mindfulness predicts less stress reactivity to suppression. J Behav Ther Exp Psychiatry 2014;45(1):57–66.

18. Grossman P, Niemann L, Schmidt S, et al. Mindfulness-based stress reduction and health benefits. J Psychosom Res 2004;57(1):35–43.

19. Grossman P, Tiefenthaler-Gilmer U, Raysz A, et al. Mindfulness training as an intervention for fibromyalgia: evidence of postintervention and 3-year follow-up benefits in well-being. Psychother Psychosom 2007;76(4):226–33.

20. Godfrin KA, van Heeringen C. The effects of mindfulness-based cognitive therapy on recurrence of depressive episodes, mental health and quality of life: a randomized controlled study. Behav Res Ther 2010;48(8):738–46.

21. Ledesma D, Kumano H. Mindfulness-based stress reduction and cancer: a meta-analysis. Psychooncology 2009;18(6):571–9.

22. Xu W, Jia K, Liu X, et al. The effects of mindfulness training on emotional health in Chinese long-term male prison inmates. Mindfulness 2016;7(5):1044–51.

23. Brown KW, Ryan RM, Creswell JD. Mindfulness: theoretical foundations and evidence for its salutary effects. Psychol Inq 2007;18(4):211–37.

24. Curtiss J, Klemanski DH, Andrews L, et al. The conditional process model of mindfulness and emotion regulation: an empirical test. J Affect Disord 2017; 212:93–100.

25. Linehan M. Cognitive-behavioral treatment of borderline personality disorder. New York: Guilford Press; 1993. Diagnosis and treatment of mental disorders.

26. Hayes SC, Wilson KG. Acceptance and commitment therapy: altering the verbal support for experiential avoidance. Behav Anal 1994;17(2):289–303.

27. Boswell JF, Anderson LM, Barlow DH. An idiographic analysis of change processes in the unified transdiagnostic treatment of depression. J Consult Clin Psychol 2014;82(6):1060–71.

28. Chiesa A, Malinowski P. Mindfulness-based approaches: are they all the same? J Clin Psychol 2011;67(4):404–24.

29. Hofmann SG, Sawyer AT, Fang A. The empirical status of the "new wave" of cognitive behavioral therapy. Psychiatr Clin North Am 2010;33(3):701–10.

30. Hofmann SG, Asmundson GJG, Beck AT. The science of cognitive therapy. Behav Ther 2013;44(2):199–212.

31. Hayes SC, Hofmann SG. The third wave of CBT and the rise of process-based care. World Psychiatry, in press.

32. Hofmann SG, Hayes SC. Process-based CBT: core competencies of behavioral and cognitive therapies. Oakland (CA): New Harbinger; 2017.

33. Kabat-Zinn J, Massion AO, Kristeller J, et al. Effectiveness of a meditation-based stress reduction program in the treatment of anxiety disorders. Am J Psychiatry 1992;149(7):936–43.

34. Bishop SR. Mindfulness: a proposed operational definition. Clin Psychol Sci Pract 2004;11(3):230–41.

35. Kabat-Zinn J. Mindfulness-based interventions in context: past, present, and future. Clin Psychol Sci Pract 2003;10(2):144–56.

36. Allen NB, Chambers R, Knight W, Melbourne Academic Mindfulness Interest Group. Mindfulness-based psychotherapies: a review of conceptual foundations, empirical evidence and practical considerations. Aust N Z J Psychiatry 2006; 40(4):285–94.

37. Killingsworth MA, Gilbert DT. A wandering mind is an unhappy mind. Science 2010;330(6006):932.

38. Bargh JA, Chartrand TL. The unbearable automaticity of being. Am Psychol 1999; 54(7):462–79.

39. Kang Y, Gruber J, Gray JR. Mindfulness and de-automatization. Emot Rev 2013; 5(2):192–201.

40. Wilson TD, Reinhard DA, Westgate EC, et al. Just think: the challenges of the disengaged mind. Science 2014;345(6192):75–7.

41. Brown KW, Ryan RM. The benefits of being present: mindfulness and its role in psychological well-being. J Pers Soc Psychol 2003;84(4):822–48.

42. Bodhi B. What does mindfulness really mean? A canonical perspective. Contemporary Buddhism 2011;12(1):19–39.

43. Ludwig DS, Kabat-Zinn J. Mindfulness in medicine. JAMA 2008;300(11):1350–2.

44. Kabat-Zinn J, Chapman-Waldrop A. Compliance with an outpatient stress reduction program: rates and predictors of program completion. J Behav Med 1988; 11(4):333–52.

45. Baer RA. Mindfulness training as a clinical intervention: a conceptual and empirical review. Clin Psychol Sci Pract 2003;10(2):125–43.

46. Hoge EA, Bui E, Marques L, et al. Randomized controlled trial of mindfulness meditation for generalized anxiety disorder: effects on anxiety and stress reactivity. J Clin Psychiatry 2013;74(8):786–92.

47. Bohlmeijer E, Prenger R, Taal E, et al. The effects of mindfulness-based stress reduction therapy on mental health of adults with a chronic medical disease: a meta-analysis. J Psychosom Res 2010;68(6):539–44.

48. Fjorback LO, Arendt M, Ornbol E, et al. Mindfulness-based stress reduction and mindfulness-based cognitive therapy: a systematic review of randomized controlled trials. Acta Psychiatr Scand 2011;124(2):102–19.

49. Bowen S, Witkiewitz K, Clifasefi SL, et al. Relative efficacy of mindfulness-based relapse prevention, standard relapse prevention, and treatment as usual for substance use disorders: a randomized clinical trial. JAMA Psychiatry 2014;71(5): 547–56.

50. Carson JW, Carson KM, Gil KM, et al. Mindfulness-based relationship enhancement. Behav Ther 2004;35(3):471–94.

51. Mason AE, Epel ES, Kristeller J, et al. Effects of a mindfulness-based intervention on mindful eating, sweets consumption, and fasting glucose levels in obese adults: data from the SHINE randomized controlled trial. J Behav Med 2016; 39(2):201–13.

52. Shahar B, Britton WB, Sbarra DA, et al. Mechanisms of change in mindfulness-based cognitive therapy for depression: preliminary evidence from a randomized controlled trial. Int J Cogn Ther 2010;3(4):402–18.

53. Ma SH, Teasdale JD. Mindfulness-based cognitive therapy for depression: replication and exploration of differential relapse prevention effects. J Consult Clin Psychol 2004;72(1):31–40.

54. Williams JMG, Crane C, Barnhofer T, et al. Mindfulness-based cognitive therapy for preventing relapse in recurrent depression: a randomized dismantling trial. J Consult Clin Psychol 2014;82(2):275–86.

55. Eisendrath SJ, Gillung E, Delucchi KL, et al. A randomized controlled trial of mindfulness-based cognitive therapy for treatment-resistant depression. Psychother Psychosom 2016;85(2):99–110.
56. Cohen JN, Jensen D, Stange JP, et al. The immediate and long-term effects of an intensive meditation retreat. Mindfulness 2017;14(1):449.
57. Rosenberg EL, Zanesco AP, King BG, et al. Intensive meditation training influences emotional responses to suffering. Emotion 2015;15(6):775–90.
58. Lim D, Condon P, DeSteno D. Mindfulness and compassion: an examination of mechanism and scalability. PLoS One 2015;10(2):e0118221.
59. Mrazek MD, Franklin MS, Phillips DT, et al. Mindfulness training improves working memory capacity and GRE performance while reducing mind wandering. Psychol Sci 2013;24(5):776–81.
60. Creswell JD, Pacilio LE, Lindsay EK, et al. Brief mindfulness meditation training alters psychological and neuroendocrine responses to social evaluative stress. Psychoneuroendocrinology 2014;44:1–12.
61. Zeidan F, Martucci KT, Kraft RA, et al. Brain mechanisms supporting the modulation of pain by mindfulness meditation. J Neurosci 2011;31(14):5540–8.
62. Boettcher J, Astrom V, Pahlsson D, et al. Internet-based mindfulness treatment for anxiety disorders: a randomized controlled trial. Behav Ther 2014;45(2):241–53.
63. Cavanagh K, Strauss C, Cicconi F, et al. A randomised controlled trial of a brief online mindfulness-based intervention. Behav Res Ther 2013;51(9):573–8.
64. Spijkerman MPJ, Pots WTM, Bohlmeijer ET. Effectiveness of online mindfulness-based interventions in improving mental health: a review and meta-analysis of randomised controlled trials. Clin Psychol Rev 2016;45:102–14.
65. Dimidjian S, Segal ZV. Prospects for a clinical science of mindfulness-based intervention. Am Psychol 2015;70(7):593–620.
66. Hofmann SG. Cognitive processes during fear acquisition and extinction in animals and humans: implications for exposure therapy of anxiety disorders. Clin Psychol Rev 2008;28(2):199–210.
67. Longmore RJ, Worrell M. Do we need to challenge thoughts in cognitive behavior therapy? Clin Psychol Rev 2007;27(2):173–87.
68. Ellis A. Rational-emotive therapy and cognitive behavior therapy: similarities and differences. Cognit Ther Res 1980;4(4):325–40.
69. Hayes SC, Villatte M, Levin M, et al. Open, aware, and active: contextual approaches as an emerging trend in the behavioral and cognitive therapies. Annu Rev Clin Psychol 2011;7:141–68.
70. Hayes SC, Follette VM, Linehan MM, editors. Mindfulness and acceptance: expanding the cognitive-behavioral tradition. New York: Guilford Press; 2004.

Acceptance and Commitment Therapy as a Treatment for Anxiety and Depression: A Review

Michael P. Twohig, PhD*, Michael E. Levin, PhD

KEYWORDS

- Acceptance and commitment therapy • ACT • Anxiety • Depression
- Psychological flexibility

KEY POINTS

- Acceptance and commitment therapy (ACT) is a modern form of cognitive behavioral therapy based on a distinct philosophy (functional contextualism) and basic science of cognition (relational frame theory).
- This article reviews the core features of ACT's theoretic model of psychopathology and treatment as well as its therapeutic approach. It then provides a systematic review of randomized controlled trials (RCTs) evaluating ACT for depression and anxiety disorders.
- Summarizing across a total of 36 RCTs, ACT appears to be more efficacious than waitlist conditions and treatment-as-usual, with largely equivalent effects relative to traditional cognitive behavioral therapy. Evidence from several trials also indicates that ACT treatment outcomes are mediated through increases in psychological flexibility, its theorized process of change.

Acceptance and commitment therapy (ACT)[1] is part of a larger research approach called contextual behavioral sciences (CBS). Those with a CBS focus to their work generally adhere to a behavior-analytic theoretic orientation, and as such have a strong interest in the basic science that informs the techniques used in therapy. Behavior analysis traditionally focused on the use or contingency management procedures to modify overt actions, and did not have a conceptualization of the role of cognition other than it being another form of behavior that was reinforced by the verbal community.[2] This differs from CBS in that the most active line of basic research is a behavioral account of language and cognition called relational frame theory (RFT).[3] RFT has been an active line of research since the 1970s, when it was called stimulus

The authors have nothing to disclose.
Department of Psychology, Utah State University, 2810 Old Main, Logan, UT 84322, USA
* Corresponding author.
E-mail address: michael.twohig@usu.edu

Psychiatr Clin N Am 40 (2017) 751–770
http://dx.doi.org/10.1016/j.psc.2017.08.009
0193-953X/17/Published by Elsevier Inc.

equivalence.[4] Since that time, RFT research has expanded and provides a method to study language and cognition, and inform behavioral interventions. To put it simply, ACT as described in this article, is modern behavior analysis applied to clinical issues including anxiety and depression. This article reviews the foundations of ACT, its theoretic model of psychopathology and treatment, and the empirical evidence for ACT as a treatment of anxiety and depressive disorders.

FOUNDATIONS OF ACCEPTANCE AND COMMITMENT THERAPY
Contextual Behavioral Science

CBS references a specific approach to science grounded in functional contextualism and behavior analysis. CBS focuses on the role of context in understanding and influencing human behavior, with a reticulated approach that integrates basic and applied scientific activities. A book-length review of CBS exists.[5]

Functional Contextualism

Clarifying philosophic assumptions is critical for ensuring the coherence and effectiveness of a program of research,[6] as well as understanding differences between therapeutic approaches.[7] ACT as a part of CBS adopts the core assumptions of functional contextualism, which are generally consistent with common assumptions in behavior analysis.[8,9] Functional contextualism is a pragmatic world view in that it defines truth with regard to success in achieving stated goals, which in the case of *functional* contextualism are prediction and influence of behavior. From this perspective, scientific activities and analyses are "true" in so far as they help to *both* reliably predict (understand) behavior and guide how to influence (change) behavior. This diverges from some alternate philosophic stances in which correspondence between a model and the world as it actually is would define a "true" analysis.[8]

The unit of analysis in functional contextualism is the organism interacting in and with a context (defined currently and historically). This means that analysis of behavior must include consideration of context in which it occurs. Although this single unit of the "act in context" can be parsed out into components, this is done with awareness that these parts cannot be fully understood independently, but rather are distinguished in so far as it helps serve prediction and influence.

This emphasis on analyzing the "act in context" for the purpose of prediction and influence has notable implications for the scientific approach, theory, and even specific clinical methods used in ACT. To have an analysis directly inform how to influence behavior, it needs to include identification of variables that can be directly manipulated. This perspective provides the foundation for ACT's approach to private events such as cognition and emotion. Rather than seeking to target specific cognitions and emotions to alter their downstream effects on other behaviors (eg, restructuring self-critical thoughts to decrease depressed mood and increase social activation), ACT seeks to alter the context in which these behaviors occur. This is sometimes referred to as a "decoupling" effect[10] in that ACT alters the context of relating to internal experiences such that they have less influence on behavior (eg, self-critical thoughts are noticed as just thoughts, while one chooses to engage in social activities).

Another example of the implications of functional contextualism for ACT is the strong emphasis on integrating basic science. This is why ACT is aligned specifically with behavior analysis and a behavioral account of cognition, which similarly emphasize the development of basic principles that support prediction and influence of behavior and consideration of manipulable context/behavior relations.

Relational Frame Theory

Over the past several decades, researchers have developed a behavioral model of language and cognition called RFT.[3,5] RFT focuses on the role of a specific type of behavior, arbitrarily applicable derived relational responding, as a central component of language and cognition.

Relational responding references the behavior of relating symbols and stimuli (eg, "this is similar to that," "this is bigger than that," "If I do this, then that will happen"). However, humans also have the unique capacity to derive relations beyond direct learning history (eg, learning a nickel is smaller than a dime and a dime is smaller than a quarter, and deriving a quarter is greater than a nickel). This ability to derive relations helps account for the generativity in language acquisition and the capacity to learn absent direct learning histories (eg, in the case of obsessions, "if human immunodeficiency virus [HIV] is like a germ and you can catch germs from touching dirty things, then I shouldn't touch doorknobs or I'll get HIV"). Furthermore, derived relational responding can be applied arbitrarily, meaning social cues (instead of just physical properties of stimuli) can inform us of how to relationally respond to stimuli. Many studies have demonstrated humans' ability to engage in arbitrarily applicable derived relational responding in a variety of contexts and forms of relations.[11] These features of relational behavior may account for aspects of cognitions, such as how relations can be made between any number of stimuli absent direct history or what could be inferred from physical properties (eg, I drink too much, people who drink too much are addicts, addicts are bad people, I'm a bad person, bad people should be avoided, I should stay away from people I love).

This last example highlights another key property of relational behavior, which is that they can transform the functions of stimuli. For example, previously neutral stimuli (eg, driving in a car) could be transformed into aversive stimuli to be avoided due to participation in relational frames, even when there is no direct learning history (eg, I could lose control if I have a panic attack, what if I had a panic attack in a car while driving, I have to avoid driving or else I'll crash and die). Thus, how individuals relate experiences can alter the function of these experiences; in lay words, how we think about things alters what these things mean.

As these examples begin to highlight, the capacity to derive relations between stimuli arbitrarily and for these relations to alter the functions of these stimuli may account for a variety of psychological challenges. This can greatly expand the range of stimuli associated with aversive functions, which, when combined with a propensity to avoid unwanted internal states, can lead to rigid, broad patterns of avoidance. Laboratory-based research has modeled this, demonstrating, for example, that the tendency to relate to anxiety as bad predicts avoidance behavior[12] and that avoidance of stimuli due to attempts at thought suppression transfers to novel stimuli through derived relational responding.[13]

Relatedly, the derived functions of relational behavior (thinking) can become a dominant source of stimulus control, leading to rigid patterns of behavior that are insensitive to the direct environment and consequences (eg, depressive patterns of being withdrawn from other people due to thoughts like "nobody likes me," while missing opportunities for social engagement or signs of being accepted/loved by others). This combination of increased potential for aversive experiences, a tendency for experiential avoidance, and rigid patterns of behavior under the control of cognitions that are insensitive to current context form a process termed psychological inflexibility, in which behavior is excessively guided/dominated by internal experiences at the expense of what would be more effective or valued.

Consistent with the analytical goals of functional contextualism, RFT not only provides a basic account for understanding psychopathology, but also highlights manipulable variables to influence the behavioral patterns. In addition to altering context to change what relations are derived (cognitive change), RFT suggests that the literal context of thoughts might be altered such that these relations do not have the same functions (cognitive defusion). Interventions focused on changing the function of thoughts are done primarily by shifting from a literal context of relating to thoughts (eg, "I can't handle my life" is literally true and so I have to give up) to a nonliteral context (eg, "I'm having the thought I can't handle my life. Thanks for the thought mind" and then moving on with the next activity for the day).

Relational behavior can also be used to increase effective behavior. For example, by verbally augmenting potential reinforcers for behavior (ie, values or motivational work). A behavior such as having a difficult conversation with a family member may be altered to be experienced as positively reinforcing through its participation in a hierarchical relation with values: "discussing this with my brother is a part of being the genuine, caring person I want to be." As another example, specific relational frames might be emphasized in clinical interventions, such as research suggesting that the use of hierarchical frames (that one contains these experiences as part of an observing self) may enhance the impact of ACT exercises focused on practicing psychological flexibility with cognitions.[14]

As this brief review highlights, RFT provides a basic behavioral account of language that is, consistent with the functional contextual emphasis on achieving prediction and influence of behavior. It does so primarily by identifying how relatively automatic patterns and effects of behavior are contextually controlled and can be targeted to change behavior. This provides a foundation from which the ACT model for psychopathology and clinical intervention can be developed.

Psychological Flexibility

As just described in the previous sections, the understanding of RFT provides guidance on ways to conceptualize cognition and overt actions, much like research on extinction provides guidance on how we think about responding to anxiety and fear. We can use this information to understand and design treatments. Just like how we teach exposure and response prevention for the treatment of many anxiety disorders, we can teach a set of basic therapy skills and principles, without needing to fully understand and appreciate the depth of how the basic principles function. Thus, one can learn about the following 6 processes of change without a full understanding of RFT. In ACT we call these midlevel terms, indicating that the construct is based off a principle, but that users should remember that it is a construct. Midlevel terms are easy to disseminate, but will lack the specificity of the actual principle.

The concept of psychological flexibility is the ability to stay in contact with inner experiences, allow them to be there when useful, see thoughts as just thoughts, have a strong sense of life direction, and pursue things that are meaningful. Psychological flexibility is made up of 6 processes of change that all work together. Sometimes the 6 processes of change are divided into the "acceptance and mindfulness" processes and the "behavior change" processes. The acceptance and mindfulness processes include acceptance, defusion, being present, and self as context; these processes help lessen the impact of inner experiences that make following values difficult. The behavior change processes involve determining directions for behavior change and using supported techniques to facilitate that change. Although these 2 sets of processes seem different at first glance, as one works with them it is clearer that acceptance and mindfulness processes and behavior change processes are interrelated. Additionally, a recent meta-analysis supports the utility of each process of change on its own, done outside of a larger therapy context.[15]

Acceptance is the opposite of experiential avoidance. Acceptance involves allowing inner experiences to occur without attempting to alter or lessen their presence in the current moment or in the future. Acceptance is an action; it is a way one behaves, not an attitude or a feeling. One easy example of an acceptance exercise is to suggest that one treats anxiety like he or she might treat a child who is screaming for a treat in a grocery store.

The second process is *defusion*, which is the opposite of fusion. Being defused with inner experiences involves seeing those inner experiences as they are (a sound, symbol, just a thought) without their transformed functions (what the mind adds to them). Fusion involves adding function to inner experiences due to derived relations. Instead of simply having a fast-beating heart and sweaty hands, these experiences are felt as "bad" and "dangerous." When anxiety is experienced this way, it is more likely to occasion avoidance. It should be noted that the 2 poles of all these processes are not good and bad, they are always contextually dependent. For example, fusion is useful when doing taxes, but usually problematic when swinging a golf club.

The third process of change is *self as context*, which can be thought of as defusion applied to self-evaluations. Self as content involves experiencing those self-evaluations as literally true and therefore allowing them to influence actions that are unwanted. For example, a self-evaluation of being tough may be helpful in a situation such as a race or a competition, but that same self-evaluation may negatively influence actions when in a serious discussion or in a romantic relationship.

The fourth process in this area is *being present*. This is much like mindfulness, focusing on flexibly shifting attention to relevant stimuli. The goal is to have clients be attentive and responsive to what is happening in their current situation, to maximize the potential for effective, valued action. Again, someone experiencing a panic attack may be drawn to focus on physiologic sensations. There may be times when that is useful, but in many circumstances, it is also useful to pay attention to the other interesting stimuli in one's environment. Similarly, for someone with generalized anxiety disorder (GAD), focusing on cognitive activity can be useful, but there are times when it is not useful and attention should be placed on what is occurring in the immediate environment.

The final 2 processes focus on behavior change, although note that in ACT, clients practice mindfulness and acceptance while engaging in such behavior change efforts. *Values* in ACT are areas of life that are important to the person and motivate actions. Through conversation, actions can be tied to values, thus making those small actions more meaningful. For example, if a father values his family, the therapist might say, "engaging in this exercise will bring you one step closer to that vacation with your family. Let's do this for that reason." Such a statement will make the aversive behavioral exercise, a little more positive. The behavioral *commitment* part of ACT is the place where traditional behavioral techniques are integrated. Because ACT is a behavioral intervention, traditional behavioral exercises make a lot of sense. ACT also just focuses on the role of language and cognition in such behavior change strategies.

PSYCHOLOGICAL FLEXIBILITY AND ANXIETY AND DEPRESSION

Like many forms of cognitive behavior therapy, ACT conceptualizations are function based, not topography based. ACT is an intervention for issues in which psychological inflexibility is a large factor in the disorder. Thus, a functional assessment is necessary to determine if psychological inflexibility has a large role in any particular case of anxiety or depression, but it is very likely that it would be the case. There are book-length discussions of ACT for anxiety[16] and depression,[5] and the data supporting correlational work between measures of psychological inflexibility and anxiety[17] and depression are strong.[18] In addition to the outcome studies on anxiety or depression individually, there are a few studies that used a similar protocol to address both clinical issues in one setting.[19]

ANXIETY DISORDERS

The ultimate goal of ACT for anxiety disorders is to help those in treatment function better with the anxiety (or related symptoms) that they are experiencing. Learning how to function with these inner experiences (eg, worry in GAD, obsessions in obsessive compulsive disorder [OCD]) is not a means to necessarily lessen those experiences; it is the process through which clients are able to function better. When anxiety is experienced from a psychologically flexible posture, it has less impact on the behavioral choices that are made. Thus, as clients participate in ACT, they are able to start living in ways that are more meaningful to them, partially because their thoughts, urges, and feelings have less impact on their actions and choices. As the client becomes more skilled at engaging in valued actions instead of avoiding inner experiences, this skill increases. It becomes easier to allow the inner experiences to occur and continue on with life. Via the processes of habituation and extinction, one may experience changes in anxiety responses. In ACT, this is considered a byproduct of treatment rather than a goal of treatment. This is an interesting challenge for clinical trial research from an ACT standpoint because we are more focused on overt behavioral changes rather than internal behavioral changes. However, most primary outcome measures used in treatment outcome work have a mix of changes to internal events and overt actions. Nevertheless, as is reviewed in the following paragraphs, ACT generally has positive impacts on standard symptom measures across a variety of anxiety disorders. All randomized controlled trials (RCTs) are reviewed in **Table 1**.

MIXED ANXIETY

Starting with mixed anxiety disorders is appropriate because ACT has always been a unified treatment protocol for issues in which psychological inflexibility is a core concern. RCTs have shown the utility of ACT as administered by student therapists at a college counseling center for clients with anxiety and depression,[19] in a large well-controlled RCT,[20] for children,[21] and finally in a bibliotherapy format.[22] Additionally, a Web-based intervention for college students with mixed issues also showed that ACT successfully reduced anxiety.[23] Support for psychological flexibility as a process of change in ACT exists in all of these RCTs. In 2 additional publications, Arch and colleagues[24] showed shared and nonshared mediational differences between CBT and ACT. Moderation effects for that same trial were also found in that CBT performed better for those with moderate levels of pretreatment anxiety sensitivity, and ACT performed better for those with comorbid disorders.[25]

GENERALIZED ANXIETY DISORDER

Most of the research on ACT for GAD comes from the work of Roemer and Orsillo, who named their treatment acceptance-based behavior therapy (ABBT) rather than ACT because it is informed by multiple avenues of research. Their work is commonly included in reviews because ABBT shares techniques and processes of changes with ACT.[17] In their first work, Roemer and Orsillo[26] tested ABBT in an open trial with 16 adults diagnosed with GAD. Results were promising, with large effect sizes

Table 1
Randomized controlled trials of ACT for anxiety disorders

Study	Design	Outcomes
Mixed anxiety		
Forman et al,[19] 2007	n = 101 students seeking service at college counseling center for depression or anxiety; ACT vs CBT	ACT = CBT for anxiety and depression; d = 0.33 for anxiety and 0.66 for depression both groups; 55% responders for anxiety and 61.2% for depression both groups
Arch et al, 2012	n = 128 adults; ACT vs CBT	All outcomes similar at post; ACT>CBT on CSR at 6 and 12 mo FU (d > 1); CBT>ACT on QOL at 12-mo FU (d = 0.42)
Hancock et al,[21] 2016	n = 193 children, ACT vs CBT vs WL	ACT = CBT, both>WL; Large pre-post d for ACT and CBT
Ritzert et al,[22] 2016	n = 503 adults received ACT self-help book or WL; pre, post, between conditions; 6-mo and 9-mo FU on treatment only	BAI: ACT>WL pre to post; 28% post responder and 31% at 9-mo FU
Generalized anxiety disorder		
Roemer et al,[27] 2008	n = 31 adults; ABBT vs WL; FU at 3 and 9 mo	PSWQ: ABBT>WL, d = 1.02; at post 76% in ABBT vs 16% in WL did not meet criteria for GAD
Wetherell et al,[29] 2011	n = 21 older adults (M age = 70); ACT vs CBT	Feasibility study and no between group comparisons; ACT: PSWQ Pre = 69, post = 54
Hayes-Skelton et al,[28] 2013	n = 81 adults; ABBT vs applied relaxation	ABBT = applied relaxation; 63%–80% responders in ABBT, 60%–78% responders in applied relaxation
Avdagic et al,[30] 2014	51 adults; group ACT vs group CBT	ACT>CBT; d = 0.79; 79% responders ACT, 49% CBT
Dahlin et al,[31] 2016	n = 103 adults; Internet delivered ABBT vs WL	ABBT>WL; d = 0.7–0.98
Panic disorder		
Gloster et al,[35] 2015	n = 43 previous treatment nonresponders; ACT vs WL	ACT vs WL d = 0.72
Social anxiety disorder		
England et al,[46] 2012	n = 45 adults; nongeneralized SAD; exposure from ACT rationale vs exposure from habituation rationale	ACT>habituation model on responder rates, 100% ACT and 83% habituation
Kocovski et al,[47] 2013	n = 137; MAGT vs CBGT vs WL	MAGT = CBGT; both >WL; 32% MAGT and CBGT CSC
Rostami et al,[45] 2014	n = 40 middle school students with learning disability	ACT>WL; Anxiety Scale ACT: 22 pre, 12 post; WL: 23 pre; 20 post
Yadegari et al,[43] 2014	n = 16, 18–20 y old; ACT vs WL	ACT>WL; SPAI: ACT 134 pre, 57 post; WL 148 pre, 149 post

(continued on next page)

Table 1
(continued)

Study	Design	Outcomes
Craske et al,[44] 2014	n = 87; ACT vs CBT vs WL, Assessments at pre, post, 6 mo, and 12 mo	ACT = CBT, both >WL; response rates post 52% CBT, 41% ACT, 6-mo FU 57% CBT, 53% ACT, 12 mo FU 40% CBT, 41% ACT
Obsessive compulsive disorder		
Twohig et al,[52] 2010	n = 79 adults; ACT vs PRT	Response rates: ACT post = 46%–56%, FU = 46%–66%; PRT post = 13%–18%, FU = 16%–18%
Yaghoob et al,[83] 2013	n = 27; ACT vs SSRI vs combination	ACT>SSRI; ACT = combination; CSC ACT = 44, combination = 40, SSRI = 12.5
Baghooli et al,[54] 2014	n = 90, ACT vs clomipramine vs ACT + clomipramine	ACT>clomipramine, combination = ACT; ACT Y-BOCS pre = 24, post 14, FU 11
Esfahani et al,[55] 2015	n = 60 adults; ACT vs TPT vs NT	ACT>TPT and NT; ACT Y-BOCS pre 29, post 14, FU 16
Health anxiety		
Eilenberg et al,[58] 2016	n = 126 adults; ACT vs WL	ACT>WL; d = .89

Abbreviations: ABBT, acceptance-based behavior therapy; ACT, acceptance and commitment therapy; CBGT, cognitive therapy group treatment; CBT, cognitive behavioral therapy; CSC, clinically significant change; CSR, clinical severity rating; d, Cohen d; FU, follow-up; GAD, generalized anxiety disorder; MAGT, mindfulness and acceptance-based group therapy; NT, narrative therapy; PRT, progressive relaxation training; PSWQ, Penn state worry questionnaire; QOL, quality of life; SAD, social anxiety disorder; SPAI, social phobia anxiety inventory; SSRI, selective serotonin reuptake inhibitor; TPT, time perspectives therapy; WL, waitlist; Y-BOCS, Yale-Brown Obsessive Compulsive Scale.

at post and follow-up with 75% responders at post and 50% at follow-up. These investigators went on to test their treatment in 2 RCTs; one against a waitlist (WL)[27] and one against an active control condition.[28] More specific ACT protocols have been tested with older adults,[29] against a CBT protocol,[30] and delivered via a Web site with therapist support.[31] Process-of-change publications support session-by-session changes in acceptance of internal experiences and engagement in valued actions for ABBT for GAD.[32] Similarly, experiential avoidance and psychological flexibility mediated outcomes in ABBT and applied relaxation for GAD.[33]

PANIC DISORDER

In a unique open trial, the utility of exposure exercises done from an ACT standpoint were tested with 11 adults diagnosed with panic disorder.[34] Each adult participated in 4 sessions of ACT, then 6 sessions of self-guided exposure exercises. They were asked to use only the ACT training they had received to guide their exposure work. A significant decrease in panic disorder was seen after the first 4 sessions, with additional significant gains found in the following 6 sessions. Eight of the 11 participants were considered responders. A full RCT (ACT vs WL) was conducted with 43 adults who were nonresponders to previous treatments for panic disorder.[35] The between group effect size was d = 0.72 for panic and d = 0.89 for general functioning. Large effect sizes were also seen for psychological flexibility. Finally, response rates for the ACT condition were 70% at posttreatment and 80% at 6-month follow-up for panic disorder symptoms.

SOCIAL ANXIETY DISORDER

A study so small (n = 11) that randomization could not be used showed equivalent results for group ACT and group CBT.[36] In addition, there have been 4 open trials evaluating ACT in a face-to-face therapy format.[37–40] Furthermore, Yuen and colleagues[41] tested ACT for social anxiety when delivered through a virtual environment and using video-conferencing software.[42] In addition to these 7 uncontrolled studies, there have been 5 RCTs of ACT. Three of these were compared with WLs,[43–45] 1 was compared with CBT,[46] and another with WL and CBT.[47] The England study[46] had more of a focus on the underlying model of ACT in that it tested exposure exercises delivered from an ACT model versus a habituation model. The study by Craske and colleagues[44] was quite large (n = 87) and showed that lower psychological flexibility at pre was associated with greater improvement at 12-month follow-up in CBT over ACT; the same was true of fear of negative evaluations.

OBSESSIVE COMPULSIVE DISORDER

ACT as a treatment for OCD has been tested in handful of single case designs.[48–51] This includes OCD in general,[50] scrupulsosity,[49] and child and adolescent OCD.[48,51] The first randomized trial of ACT compared an 8-week protocol with an active control.[52] Since then, researchers out of Iran have continued much of this work and have compared this protocol with a long list of control conditions.[53–55] Their work is interesting, as it shows the protocol can be useful across cultures and implemented with little direct training. In addition, but only lightly covered in this article, ACT and ACT plus behavior therapy have been found to be useful for OC-related disorders, including trichotillomania, excoriation disorder, and body dysmorphic disorder.[17] Analyses of processes of change supported psychological flexibility as a mediator of long-term outcomes of ACT for OCD.[56]

HEALTH ANXIETY AND SPECIFIC PHOBIA

An open trial showed strong results with a 49% reduction in health anxiety.[57] This was followed by an RCT comparing ACT for health anxiety with a WL, with positive results.[58] Two studies tested ACT protocols for individuals with school-related anxiety. In the first study of ACT for math anxiety, 24 college students were randomized to ACT or systematic desensitization delivered over 6 weeks.[59] The conditions had equivalent effects on math anxiety. In the second study, 16 students were assigned to cognitive therapy (CT) or ABBT for test anxiety.[60] There were surprising results in that those in the ABBT condition did markedly better on examinations and those in the CT condition did worse.

DEPRESSIVE DISORDERS

Depression was one of the first clinical problems evaluated with ACT[61] and one of the most studied problems since, with 17 RCTs published over the past 3 decades. ACT overlaps with behavioral activation in emphasizing a goal of increasing engagement in meaningful patterns of activity among depressed clients. Similar to anxiety disorders, the goals of ACT for depression are not to eliminate depression per se, but to increase clients' engagement in effective, valued activities in their life. Yet, ACT somewhat diverges from behavioral activation and mirrors traditional CBT in that additional emphasis is placed on targeting cognitive and related psychological barriers that may impede valued action. Results from RCTs to-date on ACT for depression are provided in **Table 2**.

Table 2
Randomized controlled trials of ACT for depression

Study	Design	Outcomes
Waitlist comparison conditions		
Bohlmeijer et al,[84] 2011	n = 93 mild to moderately depressed Dutch adults, Group ACT vs WL	ACT>WL on depression at post ($d = 0.60$) and 3-mo FU ($d = 0.63$). ACT>WL on PF at post ($d = 0.59$) and FU ($d = .66$). PF mediated treatment effects on depression.
Carlbring et al,[85] 2013	n = 80 diagnosed depressed Swedish adults, Online Self-Help ACT vs WL	ACT>WL on depression at post ($d = 0.98$) with 25% responding to ACT vs 5% in WL. ACT = WL on QOL at post.
Dindo et al,[67] 2012	n = 45 patients with diagnosed comorbid depression and migraines in the United States, ACT plus education workshop vs WL	ACT>WL on depression at 3-mo FU ($d = 1.18$) with 77% recovered from depression in ACT vs 8% in WL. ACT>WL on QOL at FU ($d = 0.69–1.03$).
Fledderus et al,[86] 2011	n = 376 mild to moderately depressed and anxious Dutch adults, Self-Help ACT with E-mail Support (ACT-E) vs ACT Without E-mail (ACT-M) vs WL	ACT-E and ACT-M>WL on depression at post (ACT-E $d = 0.74$, ACT-M $d = 0.89$) with 34%/39% responding to ACT-E/ACT-M vs 6% in WL. ACT>WL on QOL at post. ACT>WL on PF at post. PF mediated treatment effects on depression (Fledderus et al, 2013).
Kohtala et al,[87] 2015	n = 57 depressed adults in Finland, Individual ACT vs WL	ACT>WL on depression at post ($d = 0.93$). ACT>WL on QOL at post ($d = 0.58–0.64$). ACT>WL on PF at post ($d = 0.61$).
Lappalainen et al,[75] 2015	n = 39 diagnosed depressed adults in Finland, Online Self-Help ACT vs Waitlist	ACT>WL on depression at post ($g = 0.83$) with 50% recovered from depression in ACT vs 10% in WL. ACT>WL on PF at post ($g = 0.53–.67$).
TAU/active comparison conditions		
Folke et al,[70] 2012	n = 34 Swedish diagnosed depressed adults on long-term sick leave, Group ACT vs TAU	ACT>TAU on depression at post and 18-mo FU ($d = 0.86$) with 27% responding at post and 36% at FU in ACT vs 0% at post and 9% at FU in TAU. ACT>TAU on QOL ($d = 0.71$).
Gaudiano et al,[68] 2015	n = 13 patients with diagnosed comorbid depression and psychosis in the United States, individual ACT + TAU vs TAU	ACT>TAU on depression (although not analyzed statistically) at post ($d = 0.86$) with 50% responding to ACT vs 29% in TAU. ACT>TAU on QOL ($d = 0.78$). ACT>TAU on PF at post (not analyzed statistically; $d = 0.64$).

(continued on next page)

Study	Design	Outcomes
Table 2 *(continued)*		
Study	Design	Outcomes
Hayes et al,[88] 2011	n = 30 depressed Australian adolescents, individual ACT vs TAU	ACT>TAU on depression at post (d = 0.38) and 3-mo FU (d = 1.45) with 58% responding to ACT at post vs 36% in TAU.
Livheim et al,[89] 2015	n = 58 mild to moderately depressed Australian adolescent girls, group ACT vs TAU	ACT>TAU on depression at post (d = 0.78). ACT>TAU on PF at post (d = 0.76).
Petersen and Zettle,[71] 2009	n = 24 inpatients diagnosed with comorbid alcohol use and depressive disorder in the United States, individual ACT vs TAU	ACT = TAU on depression at post. ACT>TAU on PF at post.
Pots et al,[74] 2016	n = 236 mild to moderately depressed Dutch adults, Online Self-Help ACT vs EW vs WL	ACT>EW (d = 0.36) and WL (d = 0.56) on depression at post with 54% responding to ACT vs 26% in WL and 31% in EW. ACT>WL on depression at 6-mo FU (d = 0.32) and ACT = EW at FU. ACT>EW (d = 0.35) and WL (d = 0.39) on QOL at post. ACT = EW and WL at FU. ACT>WL (d = 0.50) and EW (d = 0.43) on PF at post. PF mediated ACT vs WL treatment effects but not ACT vs EW. [90]
CT/CBT comparison conditions		
Forman et al,[17] 2007; Forman et al,[78] 2012	n = 132 US college students seeking therapy with depression and/or anxiety, individual ACT vs CT	CT = ACT at post on depression, CT>ACT at 18-mo FU (f = 0.21) with 82% recovered from depression at FU in CT vs 61% in ACT. ACT = CT at post, CT>ACT at FU on QOL (f = 0.21). ACT = CT at post on PF.
Losada et al,[69] 2015	n = 135 depressed dementia caregivers in Spain, individual ACT vs CBT vs MSG.	ACT = CBT on depression at post and 6-mo FU, ACT>MSG on depression at post (d = 1.17), ACT = MSG at FU; 24% recovered from depression at post in ACT vs 27% in CBT and 0% in MSG. ACT>MSG on QOL at post (d = 0.62) and ACT = MSG on QOL at FU. ACT = CBT on QOL at post and FU. ACT>MSG on PF at post (d = 0.77), ACT = CT at post on PF.
Tamannaeifar et al,[91] 2014	n = 19 diagnosed depressed adult women in Iran, group ACT vs CT	ACT = CT on depression at post.

(continued on next page)

Study	Design	Outcomes
Table 2 *(continued)*		
Zettle and Hayes,[61] 1986	n = 18 depressed women in the United States, individual ACT vs CT	ACT = CT on depression at post, ACT>CT on depression at 2-mo FU. ACT>CT on PF at post.
Zettle and Rains, 1989;[92] Zettle et al,[79] 2011	n = 25 depressed women in the United States, Group ACT vs CT	ACT>CT on depression at post and 2-mo FU (d = 1.08). PF mediated treatment effects on depression (Zettle et al,[79] 2011).

Abbreviations: ACT, acceptance and commitment therapy; CBT, cognitive behavioral therapy; CT, cognitive therapy; d, Cohen d; EW, expressive writing; FU, Follow-Up; MSG, minimal support group; PF, psychological flexibility; QOL, Quality of life, functioning, or positive mental health outcome measures; TAU, treatment as usual; WL, waitlist.

DEPRESSION RANDOMIZED CONTROLLED TRIAL COMPARISON CONDITIONS

Several RCTs have been conducted comparing ACT with various control conditions, including WLs, treatment-as-usual (TAU), placebo conditions, and CT/CBT. Seven RCTs compared ACT with WL conditions on depression, with every study showing that ACT improves depression relative to no treatment up to 6-month follow-up. Between-condition effect sizes ranged widely across studies (Cohen's d ranging from 0.32 to 1.18).

Five RCTs compared ACT with TAU on depression, with 4 of 5 studies showing ACT improves depression more than TAU at up to 18-month follow-up. Between-condition effect sizes again ranged widely across studies (d ranging from 0.38 to 1.45). Two other RCTs compared ACT with minimally active comparison conditions (expressive writing and minimal support group) on depression. Both studies found ACT outperformed comparison conditions on depression at post, but were equivalent at follow-up.

Finally, 5 RCTs compared ACT with CT or CBT on depression. At post, 4 of 5 studies found ACT and CT/CBT were equivalent in improving depression, with the remaining study finding ACT led to greater improvements than CT. Results were more mixed at follow-up, with 1 studying finding ACT and CBT were equivalent on depression at 6-month follow-up, 1 study finding CT outperformed ACT on depression at 18-month follow-up, and 2 studies finding ACT outperformed CT on depression at 2-month follow-up.

Overall, these studies suggest that ACT is effective for depression relative to no treatment, TAU, or placebo conditions. It is less clear how ACT compares with CBT due to the number of trials and tendency for small sample sizes in existing studies, but results suggest it is likely at least equally effective for depression, with some questions raised regarding which treatment may be more effective at follow-up.

DEPRESSION RANDOMIZED CONTROLLED TRIAL SAMPLE TYPES

ACT has been adopted internationally, which is demonstrated by the range of countries that have published RCTs on ACT for depression (even when this article was restricted to English-language publications). Overall, 8 depression RCTs were conducted in Europe (3 in the Netherlands, 2 in Finland, 2 in Sweden, 1 in Spain), 6 in the United States, 2 in Australia, and 1 in Iran. An additional 5 depression RCTs were excluded because they were not available in English: 1 from Iran,[62] 1 from

China,[63] and 3 from Korea.[64–66] Results from RCTs across various countries suggest ACT has similar efficacy when adapted and implemented outside the United States.

Consistent with its transdiagnostic approach to treatment, ACT also has been evaluated in RCTs targeting more unique and complex depressive samples. RCTs indicate that ACT leads to greater improvements in depression relative to comparison conditions for depressed individuals with comorbid migraines,[67] with comorbid psychosis,[68] caregivers of family members with dementia,[69] and individuals on long-term sick leave.[70] Another RCT[71] found equivalent effects for ACT relative to TAU among individuals with comorbid alcohol and depressive disorders, although it is worth noting that the ACT condition led to less required treatment before discharge from the inpatient unit (ie, greater treatment efficiency). The vast majority of RCTs have focused on adult samples, but ACT has also been found to be effective in treating adolescents with depression in 2 RCTs. Additional open trials have found ACT to produce improvements over time with depression in unique/complex samples including comorbid depression and social anxiety disorder,[38] comorbid depression and obesity,[72] and depressed veterans in the United States.[73] Overall, these studies suggest ACT is a promising approach to apply to specific depressed populations, including those struggling with comorbid psychological or behavioral health challenges.

DEPRESSION RANDOMIZED CONTROLLED TRIAL TREATMENT FORMATS

Individual (one-on-one) therapy is the most common treatment format ACT has been evaluated in for depression, with a total of 7 RCTs. These studies found ACT outperforms WL, TAU, and a minimal support group, with largely equivalent effects relative to CT/CBT. Among studies reporting rates, ACT response rates ranged from 50% to 58%, with depression recovery rates ranging from 24% to 82%.

ACT has also been evaluated in 6 RCTs in a group format, one of which used a single-day workshop format.[67] These studies similarly found ACT outperforms WL and TAU, with equivalent or greater outcomes relative to CT. ACT response rates ranged between 27% and 36% in the one study reporting reliable change,[70] and 77% recovered from depression in ACT at 3-month follow-up after a 1-day workshop.[67]

Four RCTs evaluated ACT in a self-help format for depression, with 3 using an online delivery format and 1 testing a self-help book with e-mail support. These studies almost exclusively compared ACT with WL, finding that ACT produces significant improvements in depression relative to no treatment at post and up to 6-month follow-up with effect sizes ranging between Cohen's d of 0.32 and 0.98. ACT delivered online also outperformed an active comparison condition of expressive writing at post, although both conditions had equivalent positive effects on depression at follow-up.[74] Response rates from ACT varied between 25% and 54%, with one study finding that 50% recovered from depression following an ACT self-help program.[75]

One additional RCT, excluded from the table because it did not include a non-ACT condition, compared ACT delivered through an online program (with minimal therapist contact) versus face-to-face therapy among 38 depressed adults from Finland.[76] Participants receiving an online program actually demonstrated stronger improvements at 6-month follow-up on depressive symptoms ($g = 0.76$) and life satisfaction ($g = 0.75$) relative to face-to-face ACT. Although whether ACT consistently leads to larger effects in online formats is questionable and requires further study, these results at least suggest that ACT can be delivered in an online format with similar impact on depression.

Overall, these studies indicate that ACT is effective across a variety of modalities for depression, including individual therapy, group therapy, and self-help. These include formats that are especially promising for increasing the reach of services in cost-effective formats, such as 1-day workshops, self-help books, and Web sites. This is consistent with a recent review of treatments for depression in which recommendations were made to focus research efforts on such cost-effective methods for expanding depression services.[77]

DEPRESSION RANDOMIZED CONTROLLED TRIAL OUTCOMES WITH POSITIVE MENTAL HEALTH AND QUALITY OF LIFE

Although showing ACT reduces depressive symptoms helps demonstrate its relevance for depressed populations, it is important to also consider whether this treatment improves positive mental health and quality of life, which are also important outcomes that fit particularly well with the goals of ACT. Nine of the 17 RCTs evaluated the impact of treatment on quality of life (including quality of life, positive mental health, and/or functioning). ACT improved quality of life relative to WL in 4 of 5 trials with Cohen's d effect sizes ranging between 0.39 and 1.03, up to 3-month follow-up. ACT also improved quality of life relative to TAU in 2 trials ($d = 0.71–0.78$), expressive writing in 1 trial ($d = 0.35$), and minimal support group in 1 trial ($d = 0.62$). However, ACT was generally equivalent to CBT/CT on quality of life in the 2 trials, including this measure, with CT actually outperforming ACT on quality of life in 1 case at 18-month follow-up.[78]

Overall, these results indicate that ACT improves quality of life in addition to symptom severity among depressed samples, although it is unclear how efficacy compares with CBT in this domain.

DEPRESSION RANDOMIZED CONTROLLED TRIAL PROCESSES OF CHANGE

Twelve of 17 depression ACT RCTs examined processes of change (psychological flexibility and its specific component processes). Studies found that ACT produced greater improvements in psychological flexibility relative to WL in 3 RCTs (Cohen's d ranging from 0.50 to 0.67), relative to TAU in 3 RCTs (d ranging from 0.64 to 0.76), and relative to placebo conditions (expressive writing $d = 0.43$, minimal support group $d = 0.77$). However, only 2 of 4 RCTs found that ACT improved psychological flexibility relative to CT/CBT, with the other 2 studies finding equal improvements between conditions.

Formal mediational analyses in 3 RCTs indicated that changes in psychological flexibility mediated the impact of ACT relative to WL on depression. One additional study found through formal mediational analyses that cognitive defusion mediated the impact of ACT versus CT on depression.[79]

Overall, these results indicate that ACT appears to effectively target its key mechanism of change, psychological flexibility, and that improvements in psychological flexibility mediate treatment outcomes with most comparison conditions. However, the differential impact of ACT on psychological inflexibility relative to CT/CBT is inconsistent and somewhat unclear based on the existing literature.

SUMMARY

The goal for this article was to present the model from which ACT research occurs as well as provide an exhaustive list of all published work on ACT for anxiety disorders and depression, as ACT is a unified treatment protocol and there are a growing number of trials testing ACT across anxiety and depression issues. This base of knowledge provides initial support for ACT. There is a larger amount of work on ACT for GAD, social anxiety, and OCD. The work in panic disorder and health anxiety is in its infancy; there has been very little with specific phobias. However, there is also a large amount of research indicating ACT is effective for depression, and potentially as effective as traditional CBT.

After an earlier debate about the differences and similarities between ACT and more traditional CBT,[80] ACT is now generally considered part of a new generation of CBT approaches focused on process-based treatments.[81,82] As one of the modern CBTs, there are a number of areas for future research with ACT (eg, optimizing dissemination and implementation, studying mechanisms of change, moderators). For example, there is a need to clarify which clients might benefit more from traditional CBT or ACT within the depression and anxiety disorders. This may be particularly true for anxiety disorders in which the current research is fairly limited with some specific disorders and further work is needed to clarify the potential efficacy of ACT and treatment-matching factors. Overall, ACT's evidence base for depressive and anxiety disorders continues to grow, indicating this unique, modern CBT is a promising treatment approach warranting dissemination and further study.

REFERENCES

1. Hayes SC, Strosahl KD, Wilson KG. Acceptance and commitment therapy: the process and practice of mindful change. 2nd edition. New York: Guilford Press; 2012.
2. Skinner BF. Verbal behavior. East Norwalk (CT): Appleton-Century-Crofts; 1957.
3. Hayes SC, Barnes-Holmes D, Roche B. Relational frame theory: a post-Skinnerian account of human language and cognition. New York: Kluwer Academic/Plenum Publishers; 2001.
4. Dougher M, Twohig MP, Madden GJ. Editorial: Basic and translational research on stimulus–stimulus relations. J Exp Anal Behav 2014;101(1):1–9.
5. Zettle RD, Hayes SC, Barnes-Holmes D, et al. The Wiley handbook of contextual behavioral science. Chichester (West Sussex, UK): Wiley-Blackwell; 2016.
6. Hayes SC, Long DM, Levin ME, et al. Treatment development: can we find a better way? Clin Psychol Rev 2013;33(7):870–82.
7. Hayes SC, Levin ME, Plumb-Vilardaga J, et al. Acceptance and commitment therapy and contextual behavioral science: Examining the progress of a distinctive model of behavioral and cognitive therapy. Behav Ther 2013;44(2):180–98.
8. Hayes SC, Hayes LJ, Reese HW. Finding the philosophical core: a review of Stephen C. Pepper's World Hypotheses: a study in evidence. J Exp Anal Behav 1988;50(1):97–111.
9. Hayes SC, Barnes-Holmes D, Wilson KG. Contextual behavioral science: creating a science more adequate to the challenge of the human condition. J Contextual Behav Sci 2012;1(1):1–16.
10. Levin ME, Luoma JB, Haeger JA. Decoupling as a mechanism of change in mindfulness and acceptance: a literature review. Behav Modif 2015;39(6):870–911.
11. De Houwer J, Dymond S, Roche B. Advances in relational frame theory: research and application. Oakland (CA): New Harbinger Publications; 2013.
12. Levin ME, Haeger J, Smith GS. Examining the role of implicit emotional judgments in social anxiety and experiential avoidance. Journal of Psychopathology and Behavioral Assessment 2017;39(2):264–78.

13. Hooper N, Sandoz EK, Ashton J, et al. Comparing thought suppression and acceptance as coping techniques for food cravings. Eat Behav 2012;13(1):62–4.

14. Foody M, Barnes-Holmes Y, Barnes-Holmes D, et al. An empirical investigation of the role of self, hierarchy, and distinction in a common act exercise. Psychol Rec 2015;65(2):231–43.

15. Levin ME, Hildebrandt MJ, Lillis J, et al. The impact of treatment components suggested by the psychological flexibility model: a meta-analysis of laboratory-based component studies. Behav Ther 2012;43(4):741–56.

16. Eifert GH, Forsyth JP. Acceptance and commitment therapy for anxiety disorders: a practitioner's treatment guide to using mindfulness, acceptance, and values-based behavior change strategies. Oakland (CA): New Harbinger Publications; 2005.

17. Bluett EJ, Homan KJ, Morrison KL, et al. Acceptance and commitment therapy for anxiety and OCD spectrum disorders: An empirical review. J Anxiety Disord 2014;28(6):612–24.

18. Ruiz FJ. A review of acceptance and commitment therapy (ACT) empirical evidence: correlational, experimental psychopathology, component and outcome studies. Int J Psychol Psychol Ther 2010;10(1):125–62.

19. Forman EM, Herbert JD, Moitra E, et al. A randomized controlled effectiveness trial of acceptance and commitment therapy and cognitive therapy for anxiety and depression. Behav Modif 2007;31(6):772–99.

20. Arch JJ, Eifert GH, Davies C, et al. Randomized clinical trial of cognitive behavioral therapy (CBT) versus acceptance and commitment therapy (ACT) for mixed anxiety disorders. J Consult Clin Psychol 2012;80(5):750–65.

21. Hancock KM, Swain J, Hainsworth CJ, et al. Acceptance and commitment therapy versus cognitive behavior therapy for children with anxiety: outcomes of a randomized controlled trial. J Clin Child Adolesc Psychol 2016. [Epub ahead of print].

22. Ritzert TR, Forsyth JP, Sheppard SC, et al. Evaluating the effectiveness of ACT for anxiety disorders in a self-help context: outcomes from a randomized wait-list controlled trial. Behav Ther 2016;47(4):444–59.

23. Levin ME, Haeger JA, Pierce BG, et al. Web-based acceptance and commitment therapy for mental health problems in college students: a randomized controlled trial. Behav Modif 2017;41(1):141–62.

24. Arch JJ, Wolitzky-Taylor KB, Eifert GH, et al. Longitudinal treatment mediation of traditional cognitive behavioral therapy and acceptance and commitment therapy for anxiety disorders. Behav Res Ther 2012;50(7):469–78.

25. Wolitzky-Taylor KB, Arch JJ, Rosenfield D, et al. Moderators and non-specific predictors of treatment outcome for anxiety disorders: a comparison of cognitive behavioral therapy to acceptance and commitment therapy. J Consult Clin Psychol 2012;80(5):786.

26. Roemer L, Orsillo SM. An open trial of an acceptance-based behavior therapy for generalized anxiety disorder. Behav Ther 2007;38(1):72–85.

27. Roemer L, Orsillo SM, Salters-Pedneault K. Efficacy of an acceptance-based behavior therapy for generalized anxiety disorder: evaluation in a randomized controlled trial. J Consult Clin Psychol 2008;76(6):1083–9.

28. Hayes-Skelton SA, Roemer L, Orsillo SM. A randomized clinical trial comparing an acceptance-based behavior therapy to applied relaxation for generalized anxiety disorder. J Consult Clin Psychol 2013;81(5):761.

29. Wetherell JL, Liu L, Patterson TL, et al. Acceptance and commitment therapy for generalized anxiety disorder in older adults: a preliminary report. Behav Ther 2011;42(1):127–34.
30. Avdagic E, Morrissey SA, Boschen MJ. A randomised controlled trial of acceptance and commitment therapy and cognitive-behaviour therapy for generalised anxiety disorder. Behav Change 2014;31(02):110–30.
31. Dahlin M, Ryberg M, Vernmark K, et al. Internet-delivered acceptance-based behavior therapy for generalized anxiety disorder: a pilot study. Internet Interventions 2016;6:16–21.
32. Hayes SA, Orsillo SM, Roemer L. Changes in proposed mechanisms of action during an acceptance-based behavior therapy for generalized anxiety disorder. Behav Res Ther 2010;48(3):238–45.
33. Eustis EH, Hayes-Skelton SA, Roemer L, et al. Reductions in experiential avoidance as a mediator of change in symptom outcome and quality of life in acceptance-based behavior therapy and applied relaxation for generalized anxiety disorder. Behav Res Ther 2016;87:188–95.
34. Meuret AE, Twohig MP, Rosenfield D, et al. Brief acceptance and commitment therapy and exposure for panic disorder: a pilot study. Cogn Behav Pract 2012;19(4):606–18.
35. Gloster AT, Sonntag R, Hoyer J, et al. Treating treatment-resistant patients with panic disorder and agoraphobia using psychotherapy: a randomized controlled switching trial. Psychother Psychosom 2015;84(2):100–9.
36. Block JA, Wulfert E. Acceptance or change: Treating socially anxious college students with ACT or CBGT. Behav Analyst Today 2000;1(2):1–55.
37. Dalrymple KL, Herbert JD. Acceptance and commitment therapy for generalized social anxiety disorder: a pilot study. Behavior Modification 2007;31(5):543–68.
38. Dalrymple KL, Morgan TA, Lipschitz JM, et al. An integrated, acceptance-based behavioral approach for depression with social anxiety: Preliminary results. Behav Modif 2014;38(4):516–48.
39. Kocovski NL, Fleming JE, Rector NA. Mindfulness and acceptance-based group therapy for social anxiety disorder: an open trial. Cognitive and Behavioral Practice 2009;16(3):276–89.
40. Ossman WA, Wilson KG, Storaasli RD, et al. A preliminary investigation of the use of Acceptance and Commitment Therapy in a group treatment for social phobia. Int J Psychol Psychol Ther 2006;6(3):397–416.
41. Yuen EK, Herbert JD, Forman EM, et al. Treatment of social anxiety disorder using online virtual environments in second life. Behav Ther 2013;44(1):51–61.
42. Yuen EK, Herbert JD, Forman EM, et al. Acceptance based behavior therapy for social anxiety disorder through videoconferencing. J Anxiety Disord 2013;27(4):389–97.
43. Yadegari L, Hashemiyan K, Abolmaali K. Effect of acceptance and commitment therapy on young people with social anxiety. Int J Scientific Res Knowledge 2014;2(8):395.
44. Craske MG, Niles AN, Burklund LJ, et al. Randomized controlled trial of cognitive behavioral therapy and acceptance and commitment therapy for social phobia: outcomes and moderators. J Consult Clin Psychol 2014;82(6):1034.
45. Rostami M, Veisi N, Jafarian Dehkordi F, et al. Social anxiety in students with learning disability: benefits of acceptance and commitment therapy. Pract Clin Psychol 2014;2(4):277–84.
46. England EL, Herbert JD, Forman EM, et al. Acceptance-based exposure therapy for public speaking anxiety. J Contextual Behav Sci 2012;1(1):66–72.

47. Kocovski NL, Fleming JE, Hawley LL, et al. Mindfulness and acceptance-based group therapy versus traditional cognitive behavioral group therapy for social anxiety disorder: a randomized controlled trial. Behav Res Ther 2013;51(12): 889–98.

48. Armstrong AB, Morrison KL, Twohig MP. A preliminary investigation of acceptance and commitment therapy for adolescent obsessive-compulsive disorder. J Cogn Psychotherapy 2013;27(2):175–90.

49. Dehlin JP, Morrison KL, Twohig MP. Acceptance and commitment therapy as a treatment for scrupulosity in obsessive compulsive disorder. Behav Modif 2013; 37(3):409–30.

50. Twohig M, Hayes S, Masucla A. Increasing willingness to experience obsessions: acceptance and commitment therapy as a treatment for obsessive-compulsive disorder. Behav Ther 2006;37(1):3–13.

51. Barney JY, Field CE, Morrison KL, et al. Treatment of pediatric obsessive compulsive disorder utilizing parent-facilitated acceptance and commitment therapy. Psychol Sch 2017;54(1):88–100.

52. Twohig M, Hayes S, Plumb J, et al. A randomized clinical trial of acceptance and commitment therapy versus progressive relaxation training for obsessive-compulsive disorder. J Consult Clin Psychol 2010;78(5):705–16.

53. Vakili Y, Gharraee B, Habibi M, et al. The comparison of acceptance and commitment therapy with selective serotonin reuptake inhibitors in the treatment of obsessive-compulsive disorder. Zahedan J Res Med Sci 2014;16(10):10–4.

54. Baghooli H, Dolatshahi B, Mohammadkhani P, et al. Effectiveness of acceptance and commitment therapy in reduction of severity symptoms of patients with obsessive–compulsive disorder. Adv Environ Biol 2014;8(7):2519–25.

55. Esfahani M, Kjbaf MB, Abedi MR. Evaluation and comparison of the effects of time perspective therapy, acceptance and commitment therapy and narrative therapy on severity of symptoms of obsessive-compulsive disorder. J Indian Acad Appl Psychol 2015;41(3):148.

56. Twohig MP, Vilardaga JCP, Levin ME, et al. Changes in psychological flexibility during acceptance and commitment therapy for obsessive compulsive disorder. J Contextual Behav Sci 2015;4(3):196–202.

57. Eilenberg T, Kronstrand L, Fink P, et al. Acceptance and commitment group therapy for health anxiety–results from a pilot study. J Anxiety Disord 2013;27(5): 461–8.

58. Eilenberg T, Fink P, Jensen J, et al. Acceptance and commitment group therapy (ACT-G) for health anxiety: a randomized controlled trial. Psychol Med 2016; 46(01):103–15.

59. Zettle RD. Acceptance and commitment therapy (ACT) vs. systematic desensitization in treatment of mathematics anxiety. Psychol Rec 2003;53(2):197–215.

60. Brown LA, Forman EM, Herbert JD, et al. A randomized controlled trial of acceptance-based behavior therapy and cognitive therapy for test anxiety: a pilot study. Behavior Modification 2011;35(1):31–53.

61. Zettle RD, Hayes SC. Component and process analysis of cognitive therapy. Psychol Rep 1987;61(3):939–53.

62. Dabbaghi P, Dowran B, Taghva A. Effectiveness of group training of acceptance and commitment therapy on depression symptoms in soldiers. EBNESINA 2016; 18(2):19–25.

63. Zhao W, Zhou Y, Liu X, et al. Effectiveness of acceptance and commitment therapy on depression. Chin J Clin Psychol 2013;21(1):153–7.

64. Cho HJ. The development and effect of an ACT Program based on Loving-kindness Meditation for depressive students. Korean J Couns Psychol 2012;24: 827–46.
65. Yang SYS, Shin HK. Effects of acceptance and commitment therapy on psychological acceptance, psychological well-being, depression and suicidal ideation of depressed college students. Korean J Clin Psychol 2013;32.
66. Kim H, Park K. The effects of process variables in acceptance commitment therapy for women's depression. Korean J Clin Psychol 2014;33:429–60.
67. Dindo L, Recober A, Marchman JN, et al. One-day behavioral treatment for patients with comorbid depression and migraine: a pilot study. Behav Res Ther 2012;50(9):537–43.
68. Gaudiano BA, Busch AM, Wenze SJ, et al. Acceptance-based behavior therapy for depression with psychosis: results from a pilot feasibility randomized controlled trial. J Psychiatr Pract 2015;21(5):320.
69. Losada A, Márquez-González M, Romero-Moreno R, et al. Cognitive–behavioral therapy (CBT) versus acceptance and commitment therapy (ACT) for dementia family caregivers with significant depressive symptoms: results of a randomized clinical trial. J Consult Clin Psychol 2015;83(4):760.
70. Folke F, Parling T, Melin L. Acceptance and commitment therapy for depression: a preliminary randomized clinical trial for unemployed on long-term sick leave. Cogn Behav Pract 2012;19(4):583–94.
71. Petersen CL, Zettle RD. Treating inpatients with comorbid depression and alcohol use disorders: a comparison of acceptance and commitment therapy versus treatment as usual. Psychol Rec 2009;59(4):521.
72. Berman MI, Morton SN, Hegel MT. Uncontrolled pilot study of an acceptance and commitment therapy and health at every size intervention for obese, depressed women: accept yourself! Psychotherapy 2016;53(4):462.
73. Walser RD, Karlin BE, Trockel M, et al. Training in and implementation of Acceptance and Commitment Therapy for depression in the Veterans Health Administration: therapist and patient outcomes. Behav Res Ther 2013;51(9):555–63.
74. Pots WT, Fledderus M, Meulenbeek PA, et al. Acceptance and commitment therapy as a web-based intervention for depressive symptoms: randomised controlled trial. The British Journal of Psychiatry 2016;208(1):66–77.
75. Lappalainen P, Langrial S, Oinas-Kukkonen H, et al. Web-based acceptance and commitment therapy for depressive symptoms with minimal support: a randomized controlled trial. Behav Modif 2015;39(6):805–34.
76. Lappalainen P, Granlund A, Siltanen S, et al. ACT Internet-based vs face-to-face? A randomized controlled trial of two ways to deliver Acceptance and Commitment Therapy for depressive symptoms: an 18-month follow-up. Behaviour Research and Therapy 2014;31;61:43–54.
77. Cuijpers P. Four decades of outcome research on psychotherapies for adult depression: an overview of a series of meta-analyses. Can Psychology 2017; 58(1):7.
78. Forman EM, Shaw JA, Goetter EM, et al. Long-term follow-up of a randomized controlled trial comparing acceptance and commitment therapy and standard cognitive behavior therapy for anxiety and depression. Behav Ther 2012;43(4): 801–11.
79. Zettle RD, Rains JC, Hayes SC. Processes of change in acceptance and commitment therapy and cognitive therapy for depression: a mediation reanalysis of Zettle and Rains. Behav Modif 2011;35(3):265–83.

80. Hofmann SG. Acceptance and commitment therapy: new wave or morita therapy? Clin Psychol Sci Pract 2008;15(4):280–5.
81. Hayes SC, Hofmann SG. The third wave of cognitive behavioral therapy and the rise of process-based care. World Psychiatry 2017;16:245–6.
82. Hayes SC, Hofmann SG. Process-based CBT: the science and core clinical competencies of cognitive behavioral therapy. Oakland (CA): New Harbinger; 2017.
83. Vakili Y, Gharraee B, Habibi M, et al. The comparison of acceptance and commitment therapy with selective serotonin reuptake inhibitors in the treatment of obsessive-compulsive disorder. Zahedan Journal of Research in Medical Sciences 2014;16(10):10–4.
84. Bohlmeijer ET, Fledderus M, Rokx TAJJ, et al. Efficacy of an early intervention based on acceptance and commitment therapy for adults with depressive symptomatology: evaluation in a randomized controlled trial. Behaviour Research and Therapy 2011;9:62–7.
85. Carlbring P, Hagglund M, Luthstrom A, et al. Internet-based behavioral activation and acceptance-based treatment for depression: a randomized controlled trial. Journal of Affective Disorders 2013;148:331–7.
86. Fledderus M, Bolmeijer ET, Pieterse ME, et al. Acceptance and commitment therapy as guided self-help for psychological distress and positive mental health: a randomized controlled trial. Psychological Medicine 2011;42:1–11.
87. Kohtala A, Lappalainen R, Savonen L, et al. A four-session Acceptance and Commitment Therapy based intervention for depressive symptoms delivered by masters degree level psychology students: a preliminary study. Behavioural and Cognitive Psychotherapy 2015;43:360–73.
88. Hayes L, Boyd CP, Sewell J. Acceptance and commitment therapy for the treatment of adolescent depression: a pilot study in a psychiatric outpatient setting. Mindfulness 2011;2:86–94.
89. Livheim F, Hayes L, Ghaderi A, et al. The effectiveness of Acceptance and Commitment Therapy for adolescent mental health: Swedish and Australian pilot outcomes. Journal of Child and Family Studies 2015;24:1016–30.
90. Pots WTM, Trompetter HR, Schreurs KMG, et al. How and for whom does web-based acceptance and commitment therapy work? Mediation and moderation analyses of web-based ACT for depressive symptoms. BMC Psychiatry 2016;16:158.
91. Tamannaeifar S, Gharraee B, Birashk B, et al. A comparative effectiveness of Acceptance and Commitment Therapy and group cognitive therapy for major depressive disorder. Zahedan Journal of Research in Medical Science 2014;16:29–31.
92. Zettle RD, Rains JC. Group cognitive and contextual therapies in treatment of depression. Journal of Clinical Psychology 1989;45:438–45.

UNITED STATES POSTAL SERVICE®

Statement of Ownership, Management, and Circulation
(All Periodicals Publications Except Requester Publications)

1. Publication Title	2. Publication Number	3. Filing Date
PSYCHIATRIC CLINICS OF NORTH AMERICA	000 – 703	9/18/2017

4. Issue Frequency	5. Number of Issues Published Annually	6. Annual Subscription Price
MAR, JUN, SEP, DEC	4	$303.00

7. Complete Mailing Address of Known Office of Publication (Not printer) (Street, city, county, state, and ZIP+4®)

ELSEVIER INC.
230 Park Avenue, Suite 800
New York, NY 10169

Contact Person: STEPHEN R. BUSHING
Telephone (Include area code): 215-239-3688

8. Complete Mailing Address of Headquarters or General Business Office of Publisher (Not printer)

ELSEVIER INC.
230 Park Avenue, Suite 800
New York, NY 10169

9. Full Names and Complete Mailing Addresses of Publisher, Editor, and Managing Editor (Do not leave blank)

Publisher (Name and complete mailing address)

ADRIANNE BRIGIDO, ELSEVIER INC.
1600 JOHN F KENNEDY BLVD, SUITE 1800
PHILADELPHIA, PA 19103-2899

Editor (Name and complete mailing address)

LAUREN BOYLE, ELSEVIER INC.
1600 JOHN F KENNEDY BLVD, SUITE 1800
PHILADELPHIA, PA 19103-2899

Managing Editor (Name and complete mailing address)

PATRICK MANLEY, ELSEVIER INC.
1600 JOHN F KENNEDY BLVD, SUITE 1800
PHILADELPHIA, PA 19103-2899

10. Owner (Do not leave blank. If the publication is owned by a corporation, give the name and address of the corporation immediately followed by the names and addresses of all stockholders owning or holding 1 percent or more of the total amount of stock. If not owned by a corporation, give the names and addresses of the individual owners. If owned by a partnership or other unincorporated firm, give its name and address as well as those of each individual owner. If the publication is published by a nonprofit organization, give its name and address.)

Full Name	Complete Mailing Address
WHOLLY OWNED SUBSIDIARY OF REED/ELSEVIER, US HOLDINGS	1600 JOHN F KENNEDY BLVD, SUITE 1800 PHILADELPHIA, PA 19103-2899

11. Known Bondholders, Mortgagees, and Other Security Holders Owning or Holding 1 Percent or More of Total Amount of Bonds, Mortgages, or Other Securities. If none, check box ▸ ☒ None

Full Name	Complete Mailing Address
N/A	

12. Tax Status (For completion by nonprofit organizations authorized to mail at nonprofit rates) (Check one)
The purpose, function, and nonprofit status of this organization and the exempt status for federal income tax purposes:
☒ Has Not Changed During Preceding 12 Months
☐ Has Changed During Preceding 12 Months (Publisher must submit explanation of change with this statement)

13. Publication Title	14. Issue Date for Circulation Data Below
PSYCHIATRIC CLINICS OF NORTH AMERICA	JUNE 2017

15. Extent and Nature of Circulation

			Average No. Copies Each Issue During Preceding 12 Months	No. Copies of Single Issue Published Nearest to Filing Date
a. Total Number of Copies (Net press run)			412	314
b. Paid Circulation (By Mail and Outside the Mail)	(1)	Mailed Outside-County Paid Subscriptions Stated on PS Form 3541 (Include paid distribution above nominal rate, advertiser's proof copies, and exchange copies)	172	145
	(2)	Mailed In-County Paid Subscriptions Stated on PS Form 3541 (Include paid distribution above nominal rate, advertiser's proof copies, and exchange copies)	0	0
	(3)	Paid Distribution Outside the Mails Including Sales Through Dealers and Carriers, Street Vendors, Counter Sales, and Other Paid Distribution Outside USPS®	129	105
	(4)	Paid Distribution by Other Classes of Mail Through the USPS (e.g., First-Class Mail®)	0	0
c. Total Paid Distribution (Sum of 15b (1), (2), (3), and (4))			301	250
d. Free or Nominal Rate Distribution (By Mail and Outside the Mail)	(1)	Free or Nominal Rate Outside-County Copies Included on PS Form 3541	66	64
	(2)	Free or Nominal Rate In-County Copies Included on PS Form 3541	0	0
	(3)	Free or Nominal Rate Copies Mailed at Other Classes Through the USPS (e.g., First-Class Mail)	0	0
	(4)	Free or Nominal Rate Distribution Outside the Mail (Carriers or other means)	0	0
e. Total Free or Nominal Rate Distribution (Sum of 15d (1), (2), (3) and (4))			66	64
f. Total Distribution (Sum of 15c and 15e)			367	314
g. Copies not Distributed (See Instructions to Publishers #4 (page #3))			45	0
h. Total (Sum of 15f and g)			412	314
i. Percent Paid (15c divided by 15f times 100)			82.02%	79.62%

* If you are claiming electronic copies, go to line 16 on page 3. If you are not claiming electronic copies, skip to line 17 on page 3.

16. Electronic Copy Circulation

	Average No. Copies Each Issue During Preceding 12 Months	No. Copies of Single Issue Published Nearest to Filing Date
a. Paid Electronic Copies ▸	0	0
b. Total Paid Print Copies (Line 15c) + Paid Electronic Copies (Line 16a) ▸	301	250
c. Total Print Distribution (Line 15f) + Paid Electronic Copies (Line 16a) ▸	367	314
d. Percent Paid (Both Print & Electronic Copies) (16b divided by 16c × 100) ▸	82.02%	79.62%

☒ I certify that 50% of all my distributed copies (electronic and print) are paid above a nominal price.

17. Publication of Statement of Ownership

☒ If the publication is a general publication, publication of this statement is required. Will be printed in the DECEMBER 2017 issue of this publication.

☐ Publication not required.

18. Signature and Title of Editor, Publisher, Business Manager, or Owner

Stephen R. Bushing

STEPHEN R. BUSHING - INVENTORY DISTRIBUTION CONTROL MANAGER

Date: 9/18/2017

I certify that all information furnished on this form is true and complete. I understand that anyone who furnishes false or misleading information on this form or who omits material or information requested on the form may be subject to criminal sanctions (including fines and imprisonment) and/or civil sanctions (including civil penalties).

PS Form **3526**, July 2014 (Page 3 of 4)   PSN: 7530-01-000-9631   PRIVACY NOTICE: See our privacy policy on www.usps.com.

Moving?

Make sure your subscription moves with you!

To notify us of your new address, find your **Clinics Account Number** (located on your mailing label above your name), and contact customer service at:

Email: journalscustomerservice-usa@elsevier.com

800-654-2452 (subscribers in the U.S. & Canada)
314-447-8871 (subscribers outside of the U.S. & Canada)

Fax number: 314-447-8029

Elsevier Health Sciences Division
Subscription Customer Service
3251 Riverport Lane
Maryland Heights, MO 63043

*To ensure uninterrupted delivery of your subscription, please notify us at least 4 weeks in advance of move.

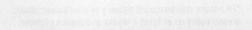

Printed and bound by CPI Group (UK) Ltd, Croydon, CR0 4YY

03/10/2024

01040390-0017